Professor Geo~~ff~~ ~~...~~ ~~th~~e tertiary sector for more ~~th~~ ~~...~~ ~~..s~~, as well as working extensively with ~~...~~ ~~...i~~an food industry. Currently he lectures and researches at the University of Western Sydney in food science, nutrition and the health aspects of wine. Geoff is the author of more than two-hundred scientific papers and books.

decoding food additives

decoding food additives

A comprehensive guide to food additive codes and food labelling

Dr Geoffrey Skurray

HACHETTE AUSTRALIA

Important Notice: Although every effort has been made to ensure that the information contained in this book is complete, accurate, and reflects up-to-date scientific research, it must not be used as a substitute for qualified medical advice. Neither the publisher nor the author can be held responsible for any reader's adverse reaction to any food additive. Neither the publisher nor the author is engaged in rendering professional advice or services to the individual reader. The reader should consult a qualified health practitioner for any medical advice. Neither the author nor the publisher can be held responsible for any loss, claim, injury, or damage allegedly arising from any information in this book.

HACHETTE AUSTRALIA

Originally published by Thomas C. Lothian Pty Ltd in 2006

First published in Australia and New Zealand in 2007
by Hachette Australia
(An imprint of Hachette Livre Australia Pty Limited)
Level 17, 207 Kent Street, Sydney NSW 2000
Website: www.hachette.com.au

Reprinted 2007

National Library of Australia
Cataloguing-in-Publication data:

Skurray, Geoffrey.
        Decoding food additives: A comprehensive guide to food
        additive codes and food labelling.

        ISBN 978 0 7336 2224 3

        1. Food additives – Australia. 2. Food – Labelling –
        Australia. 3. Food allergy – Australia. I. Title.

        664.060994

Cover design by Mary Mason
Internal design and typesetting by Egan Reid Ltd, Auckland, New Zealand
Printed in Australia by Griffin Press

Foreword

As a nutritionist, I'm a firm advocate of choosing fresh foods wherever possible. But I also know that many of the 30,000 foods sold in Australian supermarkets contain additives and many people want and need some information about these compounds.

Australians generally eat too much and the increasing incidence of excess weight and the ill-health it causes are matters of grave concern. I will therefore continue to push the case for fresh foods, not because food additives are necessarily harmful, but because they make such a huge range of foods possible and desirable to consumers. As a simple example, would children drink so much cordial, or eat so much confectionery and other junk foods if they did not contain colourings to make them appear attractive?

But even those of us who do not praise the increasing range of junk foods should have kind thoughts about some food additives. It is not long since stomach cancer was the major cause of death from cancer in countries like Australia (it remains the number one cause of cancer deaths in many third world countries). Medical researchers believe that the big doses of salt we get from foods preserved by salting and the carcinogenic compounds formed when foods are preserved by smoking are major factors in causing stomach cancer. Refrigeration and preservatives have removed the need to smoke and salt foods and so have a direct benefit in reducing at least one type of cancer.

Some people react adversely to both natural and added chemicals in foods and so need to know where these compounds are found. Better labelling assists consumers with identifying additives to which they might be sensitive, but there is still much confusion in the community about why particular compounds are used in foods.

Geoff Skurray has an immense knowledge of food technology. He is also a food technologist who does not gloss over potential problems. Indeed, in his research laboratory, he has often assessed foods and beverages for their content of additives and has spoken out when he has found levels above the legal limits. His detailed knowledge and explanations in this book will help those who are interested in what is added to foods, where the compounds come from and why they may be used.

Dr Rosemary Stanton OAM
Nutritionist

Contents

Preface

This book has been written to help Australian and New Zealand consumers find out what additives are in foods, based on label code numbers. There is also information on why, when and what concentrations of additives are used. Advice is given on food allergies, food intolerances and hyperactivity. Consumers are confronted with over 16,000 items in a supermarket and need to make food choices based on costs, nutrition, allergies and health concerns. Strict regulations by government agencies are in force in Australia and New Zealand and these are updated regularly. It is up to the food industry to justify the use of an additive and it cannot be used if there are more suitable processing methods available.

Generally additives are used to improve a food's appearance, enhance the taste, add nutrients such as antioxidants, fibre, vitamins and minerals, lengthen the shelf life or allow a food to keep without refrigeration. Health claims are made about many additives and new regulations have been introduced in 2006.

There are a bewildering number of food additives in processed foods and we need to know if they are necessary, safe and why they are used. Food additives may come from plant or animal sources, while others are synthesised in chemical factories. This book will also help consumers to avoid certain additives because of allergies, sensitivities, religious beliefs, health concerns and vegetarian or vegan convictions.

Many of the food additives listed on labels are in the form of a number code (from 100 to 1520). These are based on a worldwide system, and the numeric listing in the book can be used to look up the correct name for the additive.

Food Standards Australia New Zealand (FSANZ) do not allow all of the numbered food additives into Australia because they may not be safe, so there are several numbers missing from the list. In previous lists there were many more additives allowed, but as scientists test additives for health and safety concerns, more items are removed.

Some food additives are listed on the label with a chemical name. You can find them in the alphabetical section of this book which will give the numeric code. Use this number in the numerical section of the book to determine their safety, where they come from, and how much can be used by law.

Every effort has been made to ensure that the material in this book is accurate and based on up-to-date scientific facts.

Introduction

There are over 16,000 food items in modern supermarkets and almost 90% use some forms of food additives during their manufacturing. For many years consumers have demanded to know what these chemicals are and whether they are safe. With the advent of new technology such as genetically modified foods, many consumers may choose not to purchase such products and would want to have the food labelled appropriately.

There are often only concentrations of one part per million of compounds such as antioxidants which cannot be seen or tasted so that consumers have no way of knowing what is in their food.

Concerns about food additives have also been based on:

- religious grounds where some ingredients are taboo (e.g. pork products for Moslems)
- vegetarianism (e.g. gelatine extracted from animals in ice cream)
- allergies (e.g. peanuts and other proteins)
- intolerances (e.g. food colours and preservatives)
- health grounds (e.g. saturated fats and salt)
- nutrition grounds (e.g. vitamin fortified breakfast cereal)

- the fact that functional foods are increasing (e.g. added fibre or omega fatty acids)
- neophobia (fear of new technology, e.g. irradiated food, genetically engineered or modified additives)
- a demand for organic foods.

In the last 25 years, the Australian Consumers' Association together with other action groups have pushed for uniform food regulations that have included labelling foods with use-by dates, ingredients and the food code for additives. However the increasing interest in organic foods is not covered by these regulations as pesticides and herbicides are not mentioned and preservatives such as sulphur dioxide (code number 220) are allowed in organic products such as wines. Furthermore foods are not allowed to be irradiated during processing in Australia but almost all imported spices and dried herbs are treated with gamma ray radiation to destroy dangerous micro-organisms and their spores.

FOOD LABELS

How does the law protect consumers?

Ingredient labelling
Anything including food additives used in the manufacturing of a food must be included on a food label. The only exceptions are substances used to make flavourings, water or alcohol that evaporate during processing and water that is used in a syrup, brine or stock or when water is less than 56% of the weight of the food or water that is used to reconstitute dry or concentrated ingredients.

The 2006 Australian and New Zealand Food Standards Code states that ingredients must be listed by:

- common name

- a name that describes the true nature of the ingredient, or where applicable, a generic name for the ingredient.
- The list must not be misleading, false or deceptive.
- Ingredients must be listed in descending order by weight.

For example, reconstituted fruit made by adding water to dried fruit must be labelled as "reconstituted fruit".

The new code gives advice on how a genetically modified additive must be listed as "genetically modified", or "novel DNA or protein" or "altered characteristics".

GENERIC NAMES

The 2006 Australian and New Zealand Food Standards Code allows for generic names in an ingredient list and these are:

- cereals
- cheese
- cocoa butter
- milk solids
- nuts
- poultry meat
- spices
- starch
- sugar
- vegetables.

However, because some consumers are allergic to or cannot tolerate specific foods, the food must be listed as follows:

- Fats or oils – the source must be listed as animal or vegetable, and where the source is vegetable oil, from peanut, soybean or sesame.

- Cereals – the specific name of the cereal must be used (wheat, rye , spelt, barley, oats).

- Fish – the specific name for crustacean if used.

- Nuts – the specific name of the nut.

- Starch – if barley, wheat, rye, oats or spelt is used the name of the cereal must be used but "starch" may be listed if the starch has been chemically modified.

- Separate identification for sugars such as lactose, sucrose, fructose, glucose, etc.

Some foods such as beer, wine and spirits are exempt from listing ingredients but they must list additive codes.

THE CODE AND FOOD ADDITIVE NUMBERS

The food code numbers on labels range from 100 to 1521. They are used internationally, but certain additives may be allowed in one country but banned in other countries. For example, the yellow colour tartrazine (102) is not allowed in several countries but it is allowed in Australian foods.

Food additives are listed according to the function that they perform in the food. The additive must be named in the ingredient list by class name followed by its code number or specific name, for example, the preservative (sulphur dioxide) or 220.

The exception is specific enzymes, which are listed as "enzyme".

Are there any food additives that do not need to be declared?

A food may have different additives at different times of the year so that an ingredient list must indicate this, for example, "preservative 220 or 222", but the consumer will not know which additive is present at any particular time.

A controversial part of the food standard states that additives present in ingredients that make up less than 5% of the food do not have to have their code listed on the label. This is only the case where the additive does not perform a function in the food, for example, sulphur dioxide in dried apricots that make up less than 5% of a packet of mixed fruit.

NUTRITIONAL LABELLING

Do all foods that are sold have to have a nutrition label?

No, alcoholic drinks have a different label with the alcohol content and the number of standard drinks. Foods sold to raise funds or herbs and spices, vinegar, salt, coffee, tea and water do not need a label. Similarly, pre-made takeaway foods such as pastries, sandwiches and hamburgers do not require any labels.

Besides nutrients what other healthy food constituents must appear on the label?

Standard 1.2.8 of the Code describes the new nutritional requirements for food labels. This includes biologically active substances that benefit health. For example "Logical" margarine is labelled "with plant derived ingredients that lower cholesterol absorption". A nutritional claim may suggest a positive or negative attribute of a nutrient. Thus the label may state "unsweetened" or "sweetened" and "low fat" or "contains omega fatty acids".

Dietary fibre may be derived from plants or can be synthetic and describes that portion of a food that is resistant to digestion and absorption in the gastrointestinal tract and promotes laxation or changes blood glucose levels or reduces cholesterol in the blood. A food that contains no fibre must have a zero listed as the fibre content. "Unavailable carbohydrate" does not include dietary fibre.

Polyunsaturated fats means that there is more than one double bond in the fatty acid component, whereas mono and saturated fats mean that there is only one or no double bonds respectively in the fatty acid components of the fat.

Omega-3, omega-6 and omega-9 fatty acids are found in seeds and their oils and in fish such as tuna. They can protect against cardiovascular disease and strokes by thinning the blood and reducing plasma cholesterol.

ARE THERE ANY ANTI-NUTRITIONAL CONSTITUENTS THAT NEED TO BE LISTED?

Trans fat means that the double bond in the fatty acid is in the trans position and these fats have been implicated in cardiovascular disease (CVD). Similarly the cholesterol and saturated fat content of a food must be listed as these compounds in the diet have been implicated in CVD. The sodium content of a food must be on the label as excessive dietary sodium may lead to hypertension or dehydration. Carbohydrates, fats and proteins are necessary for energy, essential fatty acids and amino acids for growth of new tissues, muscle movements and cell maintenance, but these constituents all contribute to the energy content of the food with fats contributing 2.3 times the energy content compared to proteins or carbohydrates. Food energy in excess of your requirement leads to excess body fat.

Consumers usually have no idea about anti-nutritional factors such as trans fats, sodium sugars, starches, cholesterol, saturated fats and excess energy because they are all "invisible". They also vary from food to food depending on the processing. Our studies have found the fat content of French fries to vary from 2 to 45%!

National requirements for nutritional labelling of foods

The Australian and New Zealand Food Standards Code requirements for nutrition information panels where nutrition claims are made in relation to food are as follows:

(1) where a nutrition claim is made in relation to a food, a nutrition information panel must be included on the label on the package of the food.

(2) subject to subclause (3), where a nutrition claim is made in relation to a food which is not required to bear a label pursuant to clause 2 of Standard 1.2.1, the information prescribed in clause 5, must be –

(a) declared in a nutrition information panel displayed on or in connection with the display of the food; or

(b) provided to the purchaser upon request.

(3) where a nutrition claim is made in relation to a food in a small package, the label must include the information prescribed in clause 8.

5 Prescribed declarations in a nutrition information panel

(1) A nutrition information panel must include the following particulars –

(a) the number of servings of the food in the package expressed as either –

(i) the number of servings of the food, or

(ii) the number of servings of the food per kg, or other units as appropriate, for those packaged foods where the weight or volume of the food as packaged is variable; and

(b) the average quantity of the food in a serving expressed, in the case of a solid or semi-solid food, in grams or, in the case of a beverage or other liquid food, in millilitres; and

(c) the unit quantity of the food; and

(d) the average energy content, expressed in kilojoules or both in kilojoules and in calories (kilocalories), of a serving of the food and of the unit quantity of the food; and

(e) subject to clause 12, the average quantity, expressed in grams, of protein, fat, saturated fat, carbohydrate and sugars, in a serving of the food and in a unit quantity of the food; and

(f) the average quantity, expressed in milligrams or both milligrams and millimoles, of sodium in a serving of the food and in the unit quantity of the food; and

(g) the name and the average quantity of any other nutrient or biologically active substance in respect of which a nutrition claim is made, expressed in grams, milligrams or micrograms or other units as appropriate, that is in a serving of the food and in the unit quantity of the food.

Set out, unless otherwise prescribed in this Code, in the following format –

NUTRITION INFORMATION		
Servings per package: (insert number of servings) Serving size: g (or ml or other units as appropriate)		
	Quantity per Serving	Quantity per 100g (or 100mL)
Energy	kJ (Cal)	kJ (Cal)
Protein	g	g
Fat, total	g	g
– saturated	g	g
Carbohydrate	g	g
– sugars	g	g
Sodium	mg (mmol)	mg (mmol)
(insert any other nutrient or biologically active substance to be declared)	g, mg, µg (or other units as appropriate)	g, mg, µg (or other units as appropriate)

(2) A nutrition information panel must clearly indicate that –

(a) the average quantities set out in the panel are average quantities; and

(b) any minimum and maximum quantities set out in the panel are minimum and maximum quantities.

Typical labels

Country Maid Natural Mayonnaise

Nutrition Information

Servings per Package	12	
Serving Size	30g	

Low fat, natural mayonnaise.
Contains no artificial colour, flavour or preservative
380G net

	Per 30g Serving	Per 100g
Energy	425 kJ	1403 kJ
	(101 Cal)	(334 Cal)
Protein	less than 1 g	
Fat	8 g	28 g
-Saturated	6 g	20 g
Carbohydrate		
-Total	6.5 g	21.7 g
-Sugars	5.4 g	18.1 g
Cholesterol	6.9 g	23 g
Sodium	180 mg	600 mg
Potassium	less than 5 mg	

Ingredients: Vegetable Oil, Sugar, Vinegar, Starch, Egg, Salt, Thickener (1412), Mustard, Beneficial Gum (415), Milk Solids, Non Fat, Spices, Natural Colour (101, 160 (a)), water added, refrigerate after opening.
PRODUCT OF AUSTRALIA
USE BY: 11/10/2010

Notes:

- Ingredients are listed in descending order of the ingredients by weight.

- The product makes a claim about being "low fat", which is illegal, as it isn't.

📄 The origin of the product, the manufacturer's name and address, is required by law.

📄 The use-by date after which time the product's quality is less. The product can legally be sold after the use-by date but there is no guarantee of its quality.

📄 The term "natural" is regulated by the *Trade Practices Act* and can only be used if the product is not altered chemically and contains no food additives that are synthetic.

📄 The natural colours (101, 160 (a)) are riboflavin and carotene which are natural constituents of milk or plants respectively.

Carbonara
Pasta and sauce mix
120g
Serves 4

	Per 120g Serving	Per 100g
Energy	650 kJ	542 kJ
	(154 Cal)	(129 Cal)
Protein	5.8 g	4.8 g
Fat	4.9 g	4.1 g
-Saturated	1.9 g	1.6 g
Carbohydrate		
-Total	20.9 g	17.4 g
-Sugars	4.3 g	3.6 g
Sodium	444 mg	370 mg

Note: The above information relates to the product when made according to the stove top instructions

Ingredients: Pasta (77%)(wheat semolina), Cheese Powder (7%), Mineral Salts (339,331), Salt, Hydrolysed Vegetable Protein, Food Acid (270), Whey Powder, Maize Starch, Flavours, Flavour Enhancer (621), Yeast, Spices, Chives, Emulsifier (Soy Lecithin), Colour (160c).
BEST BEFORE 07 JUL 2008

FOOD POISONING BY MICRO-ORGANISMS

Bacteria and viruses often find their way into fresh and processed foods. The bacteria themselves or the toxins produced can cause mild or severe health problems and range from vomiting, headaches, diarrhoea, dehydration, paralysis, multiple organ shutdown and even death. However, the food industry has stringent safeguards to protect the consumer from this type of food poisoning. The codes of practice are called *Good Manufacturing Practices* (GMPs) and *Hazard Analysis of Critical Control Points* (HACCP). Raw materials and every step in the processing, storage and supermarket display are rigorously monitored. GMPs and HACCP also check for physical hazards such as glass, metal pieces and poison contamination.

The problem with food poisoning is that you cannot see these tiny micro-organisms and the food may taste okay. Poor handling of the food by the consumer may lead to multiplication of bacteria to a high enough level to cause poisoning. Many bacteria also produce toxins that are not destroyed by heat. *Staphylococcus enterotoxin* is one of these toxins. Food manufacturers label foods that have a potential for food poisoning with labels giving instructions for the correct handling, storage and cooking procedures. For example, poultry can be a source of *Salmonella* food poisoning and labels warn that poultry should be thawed or stored in the refrigerator for only four days and cooked at temperatures designed to kill this bacteria.

One of the most dangerous examples of food poisoning from strains of *E-coli* in salami cannot be controlled by the consumers so that there is no warning on the label for this type of poisoning. Recently in Australia an outbreak of this bacterium in salami caused one death and several cases of people needing kidney transplants! It is up to the manufacturer to use GMPs and HACCP to prevent this.

The most toxic compound in the world is produced by the bacteria *Clostridium botulinum*. Deaths have occurred from this deadly toxin after consumption of non-acidic canned foods that have not been properly heat sterilised. The problem is that this bacterium exists as a bacterial cell and a spore that is not destroyed by boiling food. In fact the spore "germinates" on boiling and produces the deadly *botulinum* toxin that is stable at temperatures of 100°C! Only one millionth of a gram of this toxin can kill a man! Canned non-acidic foods (meat or vegetables) that are not sterilised at about 130°C for 30 minutes can be toxic. Consumers must never purchase canned foods that are swollen and canned foods should also emit a "hiss" when opened which indicates that there are no leaks in the can seam where bacteria can grow.

Can food manufacturers make claims about the health properties of a food?

Food Standards Australia New Zealand (FSANZ) updated its health claims laws in 2006. Before this time, they only allowed nutrient content claims such as "this food is high in fibre" and some health protection claims like "calcium is important for healthy bones and teeth".

The only health claim permitted is for folic acid which helps prevent neural tube defects in babies.

The new standards are based on "content" or "actual health claims". For the first claim based on content, the wording may be "this food is high in iron" or a general level health claim on a non-serious disease such as "meat is high in iron and as part of a healthy diet may reduce your risk of anaemia". For a food to be labelled on nutrient content, it must be able to supply at least 25% of the recommended daily requirement of the nutrient.

The second type are high level health claims which may describe the function of a nutrient, vitamin, mineral or other active compound in a food and its prevention of a serious disease. For example, "This food is low in sodium. Diets low in sodium may reduce the risk of hypertension".

The claims are allowed to encourage healthier eating and boost the development of health food products over foods that have too much sugar, fat or sodium.

All claims must be substantiated with scientific evidence and, in the case of high level claims, they have to be assessed by FSANZ before the product goes on the market. One of the problems is that scientists do not know how much of a particular constituent is needed for the health claim. For example how much lycopene can prevent prostate cancer, and how much omega-6 fatty acids in margarine will prevent heart disease?

Foods such as infant formula and alcoholic drinks will not be allowed to make health claims.

There will also be specific qualifying criteria for some nutrient content claims, for example, food described as "low sodium" must contain no more than 120 mg per 100 g for solid food and the percentage of daily nutrition requirements must also be listed.

WHAT DOES THE WHITE TICK ON A RED CIRCLE MEAN ON FOOD LABELS?

The National Heart Foundation selects foods that meet their requirements for a "healthy heart". Foods that are selected must not contain high levels of sodium (salt), saturated fat, trans fat, cholesterol and excess energy from sugars or fats. Cereals should be high fibre such as wholemeal or grain or fibre-enriched bread or brown rice. The most that could be claimed is that the products with a tick on the label may reduce the risk of heart disease but of course will not cure heart disease.

THE WORDS "LOW GLYCEMIC INDEX" APPEAR ON SOME FOOD LABELS. WHAT DOES IT MEAN?

The Glycemic Index (GI) of a food can range from 100 to zero and it indicates the blood sugar levels that the food can generate. By definition, only foods that contain at least 10 g of carbohydrate per serve can have a GI; this is a measure of the rate at which the carbohydrate in a food is converted to blood glucose compared with the same quantity of glucose. Glucose is assigned a rating of 100 and other foods are then compared, based on tests in 10 volunteers. The values are averages and vary by up to 15% between individuals. GI should be used to compare foods within a food group (e.g. cornflakes and muesli). High GI foods have an index of 70 or more while low GI foods have an index of 55 or less. High GI foods should be avoided by people with diabetes who need to keep blood sugars down. Interestingly, foods such as rice, bread and potatoes were once thought to be digested slowly and release sugar gradually into the blood stream but these foods have been shown to have a high GI rating. Pure sugar has a GI rating of 68.

Processed foods such as refined breakfast cereals (cornflakes and rice bubbles) are high GI foods while rolled oats, bran and all mueslis are low GI foods. Bread with whole grains, rye or high fibre are low GI breads, and pasta, legumes and sweet potato are low GI foods.

WHAT ARE GENETICALLY MODIFIED FOODS?

Genetic modification (or genetic engineering) has been developed to produce foods that appear the same as traditional foods but have different DNA, the genetic material necessary for plants, animals and micro-organisms. The DNA material is changed using laboratory techniques that do not occur in nature. Specific genes are transferred from one organism to another. Traditional breeding can achieve similar effects, but over a much longer time span. However, traditional breeding cannot achieve the same effects using a transferred gene from a non-related species – this is possible with GM foods (for example bacteria DNA can be transposed to vegetables).

What are the advantages of genetically modified foods?

Genetically modified foods have the potential for advantages over traditional foods. For example:

- Food could have medicinal properties, such as edible vaccines – for example, apples with bacterial or rotavirus antigens.
- Foods could have a greater shelf life, like tomatoes that taste better and last longer.
- Food could be of better quality.
- Food could contain higher nutrient composition.
- Inexpensive and nutritious food, like carrots, could contain more antioxidants.
- Crops and produce may require less pesticide and herbicide during production – for example, herbicide resistant canola.

What are the concerns about genetically modified foods?

A recent forum on this very subject by the Victorian Government raised the following points:

"Some concerns that have been raised by scientists, community groups and members of the public include:

New allergens could be inadvertently appearing – existing allergens could possibly be transferred from established foods into GM foods. For example, during field trials, a gene from the peanut plant was introduced into canola seeds. People with allergies to peanuts could now be allergic to canola products that had been genetically engineered by this method.

Research has shown that no allergies have been found with currently approved GM foods in Australia.

Possible pesticide resistant insects could appear – the genetic modification of selective crops to permanently produce the natural biopesticide toxin derived from *Bacillus thuringiensis* could encourage the development of insects resistant to the toxin, making the spray ineffective. When herbicides and pesticides are used, insect resistance can occur and good agricultural practice includes strategies to reduce this.

Cross-pollination could occur – other risks include the potential for cross-pollination between GM crops and surrounding plants, including weeds. This may result in weeds that are resistant to herbicides and would thus require a greater use of herbicides, which could lead to soil and water contamination. The environmental safety aspects of GM crops vary considerably according to local conditions.

Biodiversity – growing GM crops on a large scale may also have implications for biodiversity, the balance of wildlife and the environment. This is why environmental agencies closely monitor their use.

Cross-contamination – plants bioengineered to produce pharmaceuticals (medicines etc) may contaminate food crops. Provisions have been introduced in the USA requiring substantial buffer zones, use of separate equipment and a rule that land used for such crops lie fallow for the next year. (www.betterhealth. vic.gov.au/bhcv2/bhcarticles.nsf/pages/Genetically_modified_ foods).

Antibiotic resistance may develop – bioengineers sometimes insert a 'marker' gene to help them identify whether a new gene has been successfully introduced to the host DNA. One such marker gene is for resistance to particular antibiotics. If genes coded for such resistance enter the food chain and are taken up by human gut microflora, the effectiveness of antibiotics could be reduced and human infectious disease risk increased.

Research has shown that the risk is very low; however, there is general agreement that the use of these markers should be phased out." (Stephen Leeder, *Genetically modified foods – food for thought*, MJA www.mja.com.au, John Huppatz and Paula A Fitzgerald, MJA 2000).

Ethical concerns

Concerns about genetic modification include:

- Using genes from animals in plant foods may pose ethical, philosophical or religious problems. For example, eating traces of genetic material from pork could be a problem for certain religious groups.

- Animal welfare could be adversely affected. For example, pigs given more potent GM growth hormones could suffer from health problems related to growth or metabolism. The animals themselves may suffer as well as the consumer who may ingest the growth hormone.

- New GM organisms and the genetic code itself have been patented so that life could become commercial property through copywriting.

- There is possibility of control of the world food market by large multinational companies that control the distribution of GM seeds.

Are there genetically modified ingredients that need to be on food labels?

From 7 December 2001, Australian Ministers of Health agreed that all food containing novel genetic material or protein in the final product must have its GM status identified on the package or, in the case of unpackaged foods, near the food.

This covers foods containing altered DNA and new gene product(s), its properties including potential allergenicity, toxicity, compositional differences in the food and its history of use as a food or food product. Applicants are required to submit data that describes:

- how the food crop was made, including the molecular biological data which are typical of the genetic change
- composition of the new food compared to non-modified counterpart foods
- nutritional information for the new food compared to non-modified foods
- presence of new toxins
- new allergens present.

Some food additives derived from genetically modified foods do not need to be mentioned on food labels. They are:

1 Highly refined food where the effect of the refining process removes new DNA and/or protein.

2 Processing aids and food additives except those where novel DNA and/or protein is present in the final food.

3 Flavours which are present in a concentration less than or equal to 0.1% in the final food.

4 Food prepared in shops.

Have any genetically modified foods been approved in Australia?

Since 2000 there have been 32 genetically modified foods approved for the Australian food market. These have been mainly soybeans, canola, corn, potato, wheat and sugar beet that have been produced to resist insects or the weedkiller glyophosate. These genetic modifications lead to higher yields of agricultural foods. One other approved food is a corn plant that has a very high essential amino acid content which reduces stockfeed prices.

There have been seven genetically modified food additives

approved and these are used to modify food processing. For example, protein modifying enzymes have been made that thicken cream and enhance cheese-making.

One interesting new additive is lysozyme which has been made from new bacteria using animal DNA. Lysozyme (1105) is the active ingredient in human tears that destroys bacteria and fungi. It can be added to food as a preservative.

How are genetically modified foods labelled?

Standard 1.5.2 of the Australia New Zealand Food Standards Code states that food and food additives must be labelled with the words "genetically modified", if novel DNA and/or novel protein are present in the final food, or where the food has altered characteristics.

For example: Ingredients: chicken (30%), pea protein*, water, rice, corn protein*, lecithin*, *Genetically Modified.

If a food has identified ethical, cultural and religious concerns with respect to the genetic modification, the term "altered characteristics" must be on the label because it may have different composition nutritional value, anti-nutritional factors or natural toxicants, factors known to cause allergic responses compared to the conventional food it replaces.

THE USE OF ADDITIVES IN THE FOOD INDUSTRY

Throughout history, food additives have been used by civilisations to preserve foods. The most common additive was salt and if it were not for this common ingredient, long journeys by ship could not be made. The usual common ship's ration was bully beef and sauerkraut. This sustained the crew over journeys of many months and in particular prevented scurvy (vitamin C deficiency disease) that had previously caused many journeys to be abandoned. Early explorers would not have been able to discover Australia if salt had not been used as a preservative in the making of sauerkraut.

Small impurities of nitrite in crude salt prevented deaths from food poisoning and allowed ham and bacon to sustain populations over the winter months. Preservation of other foods meant that large groups of people did not have to rely on the seasons for food, and led to the establishment of towns and cities in Europe.

Great civilisations such as the Roman Empire existed for so long because they relied on sulphur dioxide produced from burning mineral sulphur to preserve food and kill bacteria in drinking water. There were many dangerous additives used by unscrupulous merchants who used mercury and lead salts to colour food or heavy spices to disguise diseased and rotten meat. Cancer-causing coal tar dyes were also used in children's sweets.

However, with rigorous scientific research over the last 150 years, additives have been screened to weed out potentially dangerous substances. New additives have to be tested in a similar way to new drugs over several generations of mice (showing no birth defects possible) and at extremely high consumption levels (showing no changes in health). In fact if salt had only just been discovered, it would fail these tests!

Food additives are used by the modern food industry to:

- make the food attractive (colours)
- keep the foods fresh (preservatives, staling inhibitors, antioxidants)
- prevent food poisoning (preservatives)
- maintain nutrients (antioxidants and preservatives)
- enrich food (protein, carbohydrate, minerals and vitamins)
- maintain consistency (emulsifiers)
- reduce fat (bulking agents)
- reduce sugar (artificial sweeteners)

- reduce salt (salt replacers)
- affect taste (flavours, sweeteners)
- enhance flavours (MSG, ribosides)
- use minimal processing (controlled atmospheres)
- allow phases such as oil and water to mix (emulsifiers)
- form foams (foaming agents)
- form a shining surface (glazing agents)
- prevent powders from clumping (anti-caking agents)
- maintain emulsions (stabilising agents)
- hold added water (humectants)
- form viscous solutions (thickeners).

The Food Standards of Australia and New Zealand stipulate maximum possible levels of additives in food, and when there are mixtures of additives used with the same function, the sum of the concentrations of these additives must not exceed the maximum allowable level.

Supermarkets are full of foods that are safe and nutritious due to the adventitious use of additives. We would not be able to obtain many foods out of season or from different geographical areas without food additives and food processing such as freezing, drying and canning. Of course, many consumers want foods that have been minimally processed without additives and there have been developments in modified atmosphere packaging that use harmless gases from the air which can keep apples fresh for 12 months! Food additives not only keep foods fresh and therefore reduce wastage but prevent food poisoning by destroying dangerous micro-organisms such as bacteria and fungi.

Can a manufacturer use any amount of a food additive?

No, there are strict guidelines concerning the amount of additives used in Australia based on the World Health's *Codex Alimentarius Commission Procedural Manual*, which states that:

(a) The quantity of additive added to food shall be limited to the lowest possible level necessary to accomplish its desired effect.

(b) The quantity of the additive that becomes a component of food as a result of its use in manufacturing, processing or packaging of a food and which is not intended to accomplish any physical, or other technical effect in the finished food itself, is reduced to the extent reasonably possible: and

(c) The additive is prepared and handled in the same way as a food ingredient.

There is a maximum permissible level for each group of additives and where additives perform the same function, the sum of their concentrations must not exceed the maximum permitted level. This includes additives that may have carried over from raw materials.

REGULATING AUTHORITIES

Australian "watch dog"

The "watchdogs" are authorities that respond to food companies' requests for changes in food regulations or consumer complaints. They rarely have the resources to play a proactive role in researching food safety and new food additives. They rely on research carried out by food companies, the CSIRO or universities.

The Australian and New Zealand governments set up cooperative food standards to develop and implement uniform food regulations for food additives.

The system was first established under a treaty between Australia and New Zealand signed in December 1995. This system continues in operation under the Food Regulation Agreement 2002, and is enforced by food legislation in each Australian State and Territory and in New Zealand. The FSANZ Act establishes the mechanisms for the development and variation of joint food regulatory measures (a food standard or a code of practice) and creates Food Standards Australia New Zealand as the agency responsible for the joint Australia New Zealand Food Standards Code.

The enforcement and policing of food standards rests with the States and Territories in Australia and the New Zealand Government in New Zealand. Further, in relation to food imported into Australia, the Commonwealth, through the *Imported Food Control Act*, enforces the Code. There are one or more groups responsible for food surveillance charged with the task of ensuring the regulations are met. They range from individual Council food inspectors to the customs agents at air- and seaports.

The website for the Australian and New Zealand Food Standard Code can be found at www.foodstandards.gov.

International "watch dogs"

The World Health Organisation, together with the Food and Agriculture Organisation of the United Nations have formed a Joint Expert Committee on Food Additives (JECFA) to oversee which food additives are safe, pure and used at safe levels in foods.

WHY SPECIFICATIONS FOR FOOD ADDITIVES?

JECFA lists the composition and purity of food grade additives after toxicological tests and good manufacturing practices and JECFA periodically evaluates specific additives for safety.

The specifications for food additives and flavouring

agents are available and can be accessed by Internet: www.codexalimentarius.net.

FORTIFICATION OF FOODS

Processed foods may have nutrients such as minerals and vitamins removed during their manufacturing and there are regulations that allow for the enrichment of foods with these nutrients. In 2004, the Australia New Zealand Food Regulation Ministerial Council endorsed a "Policy Guideline for the Fortification of Foods with Vitamins and Minerals". This covered both mandatory and voluntary fortification of foods.

The Australian Government decided that vitamins and minerals may be added to food where there is evidence of a potential health benefit, and it is clear that the fortification of a food will not result in harm.

What are mandatory and voluntary fortifications of foods?

Mandatory fortification of food is where food manufacturers are required to add certain vitamins and minerals to food. These vitamins and minerals are added to food in response to a significant public health need.

For example the milling of wheat to make flour for bread making removes thiamine (vitamin B1) and this vitamin must be added to all flour that is used for bread making. Other nutrients are added to foods so that the general population obtains a nutrient that is lacking in the food supply. For example, iodine is added to table salt to make up for such a deficiency in the food supply.

Vitamin D must be added to margarine and oil spreads. These are mandatory fortifications of food.

Voluntary fortification allows food manufacturers to choose what vitamins and minerals they want to add to food, providing they are permitted in the Australian New Zealand Food Standards Code (the Code).

For example, minerals and vitamins are added to many breakfast cereals. Folic acid is added to many foods to prevent spina bifida forming during pregnancy.

CONTROVERSIES AND FOOD ADDITIVES

The addition of nutrients to foods can be confusing to consumers. Foods such as breakfast cereals that have a long list of added vitamins and minerals may appear to be very nutritious to consumers, however, most of the nutrients were taken out by the refining and manufacturing process and are being returned by fortification. There are over 60 essential nutrients, and most of these are not added to refined foods.

Similarly, while vitamin C is added to fortify orange juice, folic acid is not added even though orange juice is an important source of folic acid. Several years ago fruit juice drinks that contained only 25% juice were required by law to have vitamin C added during manufacturing. However, our analysis has shown that these products do not contain vitamin C since the legislation was rescinded, and vitamin C is no longer added to fruit juice drinks.

The natural yellow colour of egg yolks from hens fed on natural ingredients was the vitamin A precursor, beta carotene (160a) but artificial feeds use yellow dyes that have no nutritional value.

Similarly, the natural colour of butter derived from cream is beta carotene that the cows obtain from eating green pasture. Vitamin A is added to Australian butter to make up for any deficiency in the pasture. However in the USA both vitamin A and D must be added to butter to make butter a nutritious food, and the vitamin A used gives the butter a natural yellow colour. On the other hand, table margarines in

Australia must include these vitamins in their formulations.

Adequate dietary levels of folate can reduce the risk of neural tube defects occurring during pregnancy. This is in accordance with the Australia and New Zealand Food Standards Code that states:

(a) that increased maternal folate consumption in at least the month before and 3 months following conception may reduce the risk of foetal neural tube defects; and

(b) the recommendation that women consume a minimum of 400 micrograms folate per day in at least the month before and at least the first 3 months following conception.

If a processed food has a label claiming that it is a good source of folate it must have the following composition:

Contains at least 40 micrograms folate and not more than:

(a) 14 g fat, of which no more than 5 g is saturated fat;

(b) 500 mg sodium; and

(c) 10 g in total of added sugars and honey.

In the case of skim milk, sweetened or unsweetened condensed milk or dried milk, the label must have the following statement in large letters (more than 3 mm).

"SEEK MEDICAL ADVICE BEFORE USE IN INFANT FEEDING" or "UNSUITABLE FOR INFANTS EXCEPT ON MEDICAL ADVICE".

FOOD ALLERGIES

A food allergy is usually easy to recognise. An allergy to a food gives rise to symptoms very quickly, generally within minutes of eating or even touching the food. The symptoms are often severe, and may even be life-threatening. The kinds of symptoms that might appear include asthma, vomiting, diarrhoea, eczema, urticaria (hives), rhinorrhea (nasal drip), angio-oedema (swelling of areas of the skin) and in extreme cases, anaphylactic shock (total collapse).

The most devastating food allergy is one that can cause anaphylaxis. Thankfully, anaphylaxis is quite rare in Australia.

What causes anaphylaxis?

Common causes of anaphylaxis include milk, eggs, peanuts, tree nuts, sesame seed, fish, crustaceans and soy. These foods cause 90% of allergic reactions, however, any food can trigger anaphylaxis. The signs and symptoms of anaphylaxis may occur almost immediately after exposure and the symptoms may be difficulty in breathing or high blood pressure. The face swells up and the patient is clearly very distressed and may require immediate medical attention.

Management and treatment

Anaphylaxis is preventable and treatable if the specific food allergy is known. Parents and their affected children can be shown how to avoid food allergens. However, because accidental exposure is a reality, children and caregivers need to be able to recognise the symptoms of anaphylaxis and be prepared to administer adrenaline according to the individual's Anaphylaxis Action Plan. Adrenaline is often needed to prevent a fatality and the patient is treated with an auto-injector known in Australia as the EpiPen®.

It is important to understand that even trace amounts of food can cause a life-threatening reaction. Some extremely sensitive individuals can react to skin contact or even the smell of a food (e.g. fish). The problem that arises for consumers who may have this severe allergy is that some manufactured foods may appear to be free of the allergen, but traces of it may be present and even minute amounts can trigger anaphylaxis. Foods must therefore be labelled with a warning such as, "This food may contain traces of nuts".

A bizarre example is when a winemaker sometimes uses small amounts of the extract of the swim bladder of the sturgeon fish to clarify white wines and this wine must be labelled as "may contain fish products"!

Food allergies are usually due to the body's immune system reacting to the protein component of the offending food. For reasons that are not known, some of the food protein is absorbed from the intestine intact, instead of being digested as most proteins are. Once the intact protein is in the blood stream, it is recognised as a foreign protein to the body, or in other words as an antigen. The body produces antibodies (usually immunoglobulin E) to this antigen and the immunoglobulin binds the antigen to form an antigen-antibody complex.

This antigen-antibody complex travels around the body and stimulates certain cells called mast cells to burst open and release substances which mediate an allergic reaction. Histamine is an example of such a mediator. Histamine causes an inflammatory response in the cells that it reaches, and this inflammatory response is what causes the symptoms of the food allergy.

The foods that are most commonly associated with allergies include milk, eggs, fish, wheat, peanuts, nuts (such as almonds, hazelnuts, walnuts, Brazil nuts, cashews, pecans, pistachios and macadamia nuts), crustaceans (including prawns, crabs and lobsters), sesame seeds, cereals containing gluten (including wheat, rye, barley and oats), soy, celery, mustard and chocolate.

The treatment for a food allergy is strict avoidance of the offending food(s). Reactions can sometimes be avoided or reduced by the use of antihistamines, or by desensitising therapy, but essentially, people who are allergic to a food should avoid all contact with that food.

FOOD INTOLERANCE

Food intolerance is the term used to describe a physiological reaction to a food component. A physiological reaction refers to the drug-like side effects caused by a range of chemicals that may be present in food as natural or added components. Food chemicals that have been implicated in causing physiological reactions include salicylates, amines, sulphites and benzoates which are natural components of foods. There is also the more rare form of intolerance to food which has a psychological basis. This is due to a past bad experience associated with a particular food. For example, someone who became very sick by eating too much chocolate may have an intolerance to chocolate at a later date.

While food intolerances are much more common than food allergies, the range of symptoms that can be induced by food intolerances are very similar to those caused by food allergies. So on initial presentation, it can be difficult to differentiate between the two conditions. However, food intolerances may also lead to more diffuse symptoms such as drowsiness, fatigue, irritability, and headache, as well as muscular aches and pains.

Physiological reactions to food can occur at any age. The onset of symptoms is often delayed, and this makes recognition of the causative food component quite difficult. This is in contrast to a food allergy, in which the reaction is usually immediate; the allergy occurs early in life, and generally people are allergic to only one or two foods.

The severity of symptoms in a food intolerance is dose-dependent, and the dose can be cumulative over days of ingestion. This characteristic further increases the difficulty of diagnosis, as the symptom-inducing chemicals may be common to many foods, so that different foods may appear to cause symptoms on some occasions, but not on others.

Unfortunately, many medical practitioners have used the

safe ground and suggested that food allergies are something for alternative medicine such as naturopathy and osteopathy and not for "real doctors". As a result, a variety of practitioners have emerged with dubious schemes to test for and treat "food sensitivity". The author has been contacted many times by patients of alternative medical practitioners who say that they are "allergic" to food preservatives without having undergone any tests. These patients want to know which foods have specific additives. However you can only be "allergic" to proteins, not chemical additives!

It is very difficult in most cases to diagnose food intolerances. There are skin scratch tests and a "RAST" test which analyses blood samples of patients but the results can be confusing and not all food constituents are checked. If a particular food is suspected as triggering an intolerance, the only way of scientifically verifying it is to put the patient on a strict diet called an "elimination diet" which is free of the common allergens and intolerances. After a week, the patient can be, one by one, challenged with foods that may cause symptoms within 24 hours. In this way foods for which an intolerance exists can be determined.

When you know about food intolerance, many common patterns of illness begin to make sense. Linda Gamlin, writing about food allergies in the *New Scientist* (2005) stated:

> Evidence is growing that many debilitating and chronic symptoms of ill health come from intolerance for certain foods. The medical establishment finds many aspects of food intolerance difficult to swallow, but the main problem is the plethora of symptoms and the variations from one patient to another.

Doctors working with food intolerances report that there may be more than 30 symptoms, and that the severity varies. Some patients have nothing more than the occasional migraine or bout of fatigue, while others are unable to work or lead a normal life.

Candida infection is one particular condition that is thought by some to be caused by food intolerance. People who have this infection are told to avoid all yeast products such as bread, wine and beer. There is a common misbelief among a number of alternative health practitioners that the common Candida infection is due to eating foods that contain yeast. Candida may be related to yeast but it is a human pathogen, while food yeasts will have no ill affects on consumers despite the many tales in unreliable alternative health books.

THE MOST COMMON SYMPTOMS OF INTOLERANCES AND ALLERGIES

The most common occurrence of food intolerances and allergies are non-specific illnesses with many symptoms in many parts of the body over a long period of time (months to years). Flushing of the face, perspiring, fever and a "funny feeling" like an infection or a "cold". The illness may be transient and involve symptoms which last a few hours or come and go over many years. In the worst case, the illness may progress and become disabling.

Common symptoms include: abdominal pain, fatigue, aching, stiffness, fever, cravings, compulsive eating, headache, drowsiness, nose congestion, oedema (water retention), indigestion, flatulence, mental fogginess, sore throat, irritability, joint pain, muscle aching, sweating, sleep disturbances and diarrhoea.

Symptoms may appear anywhere in your body. They may have names such as migraine, chronic fatigue, eczema, urticaria (hives), psoriasis, asthma, irritable bowel or a neurosis such as depression.

Many consumers will have a mixture of these problems which are specific and non-specific and called "Sick-all-over Syndrome". A food allergy or intolerance may become a more severe chronic illness after several years and reports have implicated lupus, arthritis and colitis (Crohn's disease). Bacterial or viral infections often have similar symptoms to a food allergy or intolerance and are therefore confused. However, allergies or intolerances may persist over several years if the cause is not found, whereas bacterial and viral infections do not last for very long. Symptoms such as aching, fever, fatigue and headache are common to allergies, intolerances and infections. The diagnosis may be colds, flu, Epstein–Barr virus, Candida yeast infection or just "a virus". But a food allergy or intolerance keeps recurring, whereas infections are usually infrequent events.

GLUTEN INTOLERANCE

Some people are born with an inability to digest gluten present in many cereals. Symptoms are chronic fatigue, diarrhoea, bone pain, bloating, weight loss, anaemia, weakness, and sore joints and muscles. This is called gluten sensitive enteropathy or celiac disease. It is diagnosed by symptoms and a blood test. Gluten intolerance can develop at any age.

Treatment

Sufferers must have a gluten-free diet for life as this is the only treatment available at this time. They must not consume any wheat, rye, barley, or products of these cereals.

LACTOSE INTOLERANCE

A small percentage of Australians are born with or develop an inability to digest lactose, the sugar found in milk and dairy products. Many Asian people are particularly intolerant of lactose. These people cannot absorb lactose. The undigested lactose is fermented by bacteria in the intestine causing bloating, cramps and diarrhoea. Some foods are formulated with lactose, and the ingredient list on the label should warn the consumer of the presence of lactose. Dairy foods that contain lactose are good sources of calcium, vitamin D and riboflavin so supplements may be needed. However, the enzyme that hydrolyses lactose to simple sugars that can be absorbed can be purchased from pharmacies so that the lactose-containing foods can be tolerated.

HYPERACTIVITY AND FOOD ADDITIVES

In the case of attention deficit hyperactivity disorder (ADHD) or hyperactivity, "Food colouring, especially red, can make children hyperactive (restlessness, failure to stay quiet or sit still in class, talk excessively)" is the popular myth.

The myth that food colourings, also known as colour additives, cause hyperactivity was popularised in the 1970s. In 1973, Dr Benjamin Feingold gave a paper at a conference of the American Medical Association linking food additives to learning and behaviour disorders. His extensive research was based on over 1,200 cases and included over 3,000 different food additives. The work was extended and salicylates that are naturally present in foods such as tomatoes have been implicated in ADHD. The additives listed below were avoided by followers of the "Feingold diet".

Additive numbers and names

104	Quinoline yellow
107	Yellow 2G
110	Sunset yellow FCF
120	Cochineal, carminic acid
122	Carmoisine (red)
123	Amaranth (Red No.2)
124	Ponceau (Red No.4)
127	Erythrosine (Red No.3)
128	Red 2G
129	Allura red AC (Red No.40)
131	Patent blue
132	Indigo Carmine (blue)
133	Brilliant blue FCF (Blue No.1)
151	Black
153	Vegetable carbon (black colour banned in US)

154	Brown FK
155	Chocolate Brown HT
319	TBHQ (preservative, may also be listed as "antioxidant")
320	BHA (preservative, may also be listed as "antioxidant")
321	BHT (preservative, may also be listed as "antioxidant").

However, well-controlled studies conducted since then have produced no evidence that colour additives cause hyperactivity or learning disabilities in children.

Dr Keith Conners, author of *Food Additives and Hyperactive Children*, has been one of the main researchers refuting the Feingold hypothesis. In 2004, at Southampton University Hospital, Dr Bateman carried out a very extensive double blind test with 1,873 hyperactive children and found that there was no effect of either a placebo or foods containing dyes, preservatives or salicylates on the children's behaviour either clinically or as judged by the parents.

Despite this, an Australian Food and Grocery Council survey showed that 75% of consumers believed that additives caused hyperactivity. (www.afgc.org.au/index.cfm?id=129)

When I was working at the University of California, Berkeley, the *National Inquirer* newspaper tried to get me to make a comment on the suggestion that most criminals in the US gaols were there because they consumed too many food additives! The Internet is alive with anecdotal claims about ADHD and food additives with hyperactive children's support groups in many countries (www.cspinet.org/diet.html) who fervently believe that children's behaviour is due to food additives in their diet.

Food additives – numerical list

ADI is the Acceptable Daily Intake as recommended by the World Health Organisation (WHO). "No ADI" means that, on the basis of the available data (toxicological, biochemical and other), the total daily intake of the substance, arising from its use or uses at the levels necessary to achieve the desired effect and from its acceptable background in food, does not, in the opinion of the WHO committees, represent a hazard to health. Consumers who may take a large amount of a particular additive are carefully monitored. For example, people with diabetes may consume large amounts of artificial sweeteners.

100 COLOURS

Before the discovery of synthetic dyes by Perkins in 1856, unscrupulous food manufacturers used toxic metal pigments such as lead and mercury salts, which were brightly coloured, but they are brain poisons and they caused devastating health problems. They were replaced by natural dyestuffs. During the early part of the twentieth century a large number of cheap dyes were synthesised and many of these then found their way into food products.

Once scientists discovered that many of the dyes were carcinogenic, countries began to legislate what could be added to food and the number of both natural and synthetic colours used in food dropped markedly. During World War Two artificial butter was discovered (margarine), and it was coloured yellow with a substance that was later found to cause bladder cancer!

Today many countries differ in what they consider to be safe and the same dyes are not necessarily used worldwide. In the case of Norway, the use of any synthetic colour additives has been forbidden since 1976.

Professor Kurek investigated 37 patients with chronic, active urticaria and histories suggestive of food and/or aspirin-related exacerbations. Medications were discontinued and all patients received a diet free of additives and common allergens for 7 days. Double-blind, placebo-controlled challenges with tartrazine, methylparaben, p-hydroxy-benzoate, sodium benzoate, indigotine, quinolone yellow, sodium glutamate, sodium bisulphite, and acetyl salicylic acid were performed in 18 patients who became symptom-free during the elimination diet. Skin tests with food additives were performed in all patients following the prick and patch test technique. Positive reactions to single or multiple oral challenges were found in eight patients.

Information on the toxicity of all additives can be found at the University of California (Berkeley) "Carcinogenic Data Base" site (http://potency.berkeley.edu).

The situation becomes even more confusing when natural dyes are synthesised i.e. the nature-identical dyes.

What are "lake" dyes?

Aluminium lakes are made by the mixing of water soluble dye with an insoluble aluminium hydrated substrate which makes the colour a fine pigment, insoluble in water. The product is coloured either by coating on to the surface or dispersion of the lake into the product.

Lake dyes are more stable than the corresponding water-soluble dyes, producing brighter, more vivid colours and are most suitable for products containing oils and fats, or products lacking sufficient moisture to dissolve dyes.

Difference between lakes and dyes

A dye is a distinct chemical material, which exhibits colouring power or tinctorial strength when dissolved. A pigment generically is an insoluble material, which colours by dispersion. The lakes consist of a substratum of alumina hydrate on which the dye is absorbed or precipitated. Having aluminium hydroxide as substrate, the lakes are insoluble in nearly all solvents.

Regulations specify a minimum of 80% pure dye for primary soluble dyes. Most lots will be in the range of 88–92% pure. The lakes, on the other hand do not have a specified minimum dye content and typically range from 8–40% pure dye.

Pure dye in lakes does not relate to the colour value or colouring property of the lake. Since lakes are pigments, their colouring is achieved through dispersion of tiny colour particles. The more finely ground the colour particles, the brighter a colour will be. Physiologically lakes are not digested and pass right through the digestive tract untouched.

100   Curcumin or turmeric yellow or kurkum (colour) (CI 75300)

Source   Derived from the fresh or dried rhizome of *Curcuma longa* (*Curcuma domestica Valeton*) (turmeric). It is a member of the ginger family of plants and it gives dishes a mild, bitter, "woodsy" flavour and a rich yellow colour. Minor amounts of oils and resins are found naturally in the rhizome. It is often used to replace the expensive saffron. It is imported from

China, India and Pakistan. Organic solvents are used to extract the pure curcumin colour additive.

Function Colour additive depending on acidity (yellow in acid, pH 1–6 and orange in alkali, pH 7–8). Many manufacturers are using this natural colour instead of tartrazine (102) in foods.

Properties In animal models, curcumin and its derivatives have been shown to inhibit the progression of chemically induced colon and skin cancers. The genetic changes in carcinogenesis in these organs involve different genes, but curcumin is effective in preventing carcinogenesis in both organs. A possible explanation for this finding is that curcumin may inhibit angiogenesis.

ADI 0–3 mg/kg body weight

Used in curry pastes, curry powders, processed cheese

101 Riboflavin or Riboflavin 5'-phosphate sodium or lactoflavin or Vitamin B2

Source Synthesised from isoalloxazine.

Function Yellow colour and nutrient additive that fluoresces blue in milk. Very slightly soluble in water at pH 6, very soluble in water at pH 7 to 8. Insoluble in alcohol. Readily destroyed by temperatures greater than 40°C and ultraviolet light.

Properties Riboflavin is an essential B vitamin that is part of two enzymes that participate in the derivation of energy from sugars and fats. It is not stored readily in the body so that a regular dietary intake of riboflavin is necessary. No cases of riboflavin toxicity have been reported as the kidney excretes excess riboflavin in the blood. Riboflavin occurs naturally in dairy products such as yoghurt and milk and it is added to many breakfast cereals. Overcooking foods or leaving food at high temperatures destroys riboflavin.

ADI   0–0.5 mg/kg body weight

Used in margarine, dairy products such as cheese spreads, dips, processed cheese. Added to foods to maintain the amount lost in processing

102   Tartrazine (CI 19140), yellow 5

Source   Synthesised from the coal tar sulfonatophenyl pyrazole.

Function Dye or lake dye of yellow colour. Pale orange powder. Soluble in water and slightly soluble in alcohol.

Properties It has been estimated that 0.1% of the population cannot tolerate tartrazine. It is suggested that it has salicylate properties that lead to symptoms similar to hay fever (runny nose, cough, headaches etc.). Other research has shown that a few people react to tartrazine and develop urticaria and acne. The Food Advisory Committee in the United Kingdom, in a recent report on food colours (2005), stated that the rare cases of allergy or hypersensitivity to certain food colours constitute valid grounds for restricting their use. The use of tartrazine in fact is permitted in most countries including the United States of America, the United Kingdom, Canada, France, Germany, Japan and Holland.

Professor Kapadia at Howard University, Washington studies cancer chemopreventive effects of non-toxic natural colorants and other products of biologic and synthetic origin. He tested several Food and Drug Administration-approved synthetic colorants for anti-tumour promoting potential by the in vitro Epstein–Barr virus early antigen activation in Raji cells in response to the tumour promoter 12-O-tetradecanoylphorbol-13-acetate (TPA). Among

29 such colorants used in foods, pharmaceuticals and cosmetics and evaluated in vitro, six of the 10 most effective had an azo group. Three structurally unrelated colorants tested in this assay were also studied in vivo for chemoprevention of 7,12-dimethylbenz[a]anthracene (DMBA)-induced TPA-promoted mouse skin carcinogenesis. The results indicate that tartrazine is a potent inhibitor of skin tumours.

ADI   0–7.5 mg/kg body weight

Maximum allowable levels

70 mg/L in beverages and 290 mg/kg foods other than beverages

Used in   artificial fruit juices, soft drinks, compound chocolate, canned fruit and peas, gravies, sauces and condiments, confectionery, ice cream, ice confections

103   Alkanet or Alkannin

Source   Natural plant extract from either green Alkanet (*Pentaglottis sempervirens*) or *Alkanna tinctoria* or Dyer's Bugloss which is a member of the Borage family *Boraginaceae*. Blue or red powder (depending on pH) extracted from the roughly hairy perennial cultivated in China. Leaves large, oval and pointed and basal ones are stalked. Bunches of bright blue flowers are extracted with methanol and then crystallised.

Function   Very soluble in water and organic solvents. Red at pH less than 4 and blue at pH greater than 4. It has been illegally used to colour wine as it is very similar to natural grape skin colour.

Properties There have been no scientific tests carried out on alkanet. It is not allowed to be used in foods in Europe.

ADI   No ADI

Used in   soft drinks, confectionery, cakes, ice cream, ice confections

104   Quinoline yellow (CI 47005)

Source   Synthesised from methylation of the coal tar disulphonic acid.

Function   Dye or lake dye, dark yellow. It is very stable to heat and food acids.

Properties According to the World Health Organisation, quinoline yellow is absorbed from the gastrointestinal tract to only a small extent, and most of an orally administered dose is excreted unchanged. No adverse effects of treatment were seen in the two-generation long-term study in mice. In particular there was no observed effect on thyroid function or histopathology and no evidence of carcinogenicity. Quinoline yellow has therefore been approved as a food additive in most countries. Before 2002 quinoline was not allowed in Australia as a food additive.

ADI   0–2.5 mg/kg body weight

Maximum allowable levels
70 mg/L in beverages and 290 mg/kg foods other than beverages

Used in   sauces, soft drinks, confectionery, mustard pickles, cakes, biscuits

110   Sunset yellow 3 FCF (CI 15985)

Source   Synthesised from the coal tar sulfonatophenyl, 2, naphthalene.

Function   Dye or lake dye, bright yellow colour, stable in foods and very stable during processing and storage.

Properties The International Agency for Research on Cancer recommended the use of sunset yellow in foods after it considered tests in which sunset yellow FCF was administered to mice and rats by the oral route and to rats by the subcutaneous route. In the oral experiments in mice there was no evidence of carcinogenicity as compared with controls. Tests in rats by the oral route showed negative results, but the experiments were inadequately reported. Repeated subcutaneous injections in rats led to neither local nor distant tumours.

ADI 0–25 mg/kg body weight

Maximum allowable levels
70 mg/L in beverages and 290 mg/kg foods other than beverages

Used in fruit juice drinks, cordials, confectionery, Mexican spice mixes, sauces

120   Carmine or Carminic acid or Cochineal or natural red 4 (CI 75470)

Source Cochineal is a natural compound derived from the alcohol extraction of the dried bodies of the female insect *dactylopius coccus Costa*. It is sold commercially as the sodium, potassium or ammonium salt of carminic acid.

Function Dark red liquid, very soluble in water. The colour is a stable red in most foods but in alkali it becomes blue.

Properties Professor Kapadia at Howard University, Washington, studied carminic acid to uncover cancer chemopreventive effects of non-toxic natural colourants; he tested several Food and Drug Administration-approved synthetic colorants for anti-tumour promoting potential by the in vitro Epstein–Barr virus early antigen activation in Raji cells in response to the tumour promoter 12-O-tetradecanoylphorbol-13-acetate (TPA). Among 29 such colorants used in foods, pharmaceuticals and cosmetics and evaluated in vitro, six of the 10 most effective had an azo group. Three structurally unrelated colorants tested in this assay were also studied in vivo for chemoprevention of seven, 12-dimethylbenz[a]anthracene (DMBA)-induced TPA-promoted mouse skin carcinogenesis. The results indicate that carminic acid was a potent inhibitor of skin tumours. Cochineal is relatively expensive and is often replaced by other red food additives.

Properties No adverse effects

ADI 0–5 mg/kg body weight

Maximum allowable levels
70 mg/L in beverages and 290 mg/kg foods other than beverages

Used in canned cherries, cake mixes, biscuits

122 Azorubine or Carmoisine (CI 14720)

Source Synthesised from coal tar.

Function Dye or lake dye, red colour stable to heat so that it is particularly used in fermented foods that are heat treated.

Properties According to the World Health Organisation, little information is available on the metabolism of this colour. It has been studied adequately long-term only in the mouse. The long-term studies in the rat recorded only tumour incidence and survival, while many other essential observations have not been reported. The reproduction study did not reveal any compound-related adverse effects. There are no studies available on embryotoxicity including teratology.

ADI 0–4 mg/kg body weight

Maximum allowable levels
> 70 mg/L in beverages and 290 mg/kg foods other than beverages

Used in
> blancmange, marzipan, Swiss rolls, jams and preserves, flavoured yoghurts, packet soups, jelly

123   Amaranth (CI 16185) or red 2

Source
Synthetic compound derived from coal tar (trisodium 2-hydroxy-1-(4-sulfonato-1-naphthylazo) naphthalene-3,6-disulfonate), not to be confused with the Amaranth plant which is also blue-red.

Function
Dye or lake dye, blue-red pigment.

Properties
Many long-term studies have been carried out in rats, mice and dogs. Only two of the long-term studies indicated a carcinogenic potential not seen in any of the other studies. These studies were also evaluated in a report of the International Agency for Research on Cancer (Lyon). This committee concluded that because of the uncertainty about the impurity content of the amaranth employed in these two studies, the carcinogenicity of this compound could not be evaluated. The compound was banned in the US in 1976.

Several new studies on reproduction and teratology were available for evaluation. These gave some conflicting results with regard to foetotoxicity, although none of them produced any evidence of teratogenic effects related to amaranth administration. Further studies to elucidate the observations generating concern over reproductive effects have shown that, in retrospect, a study showed apparent adverse effects because of the unexpectedly low foetal resorption in control animals compared with non-contemporary controls. An extensive comparative study has failed to reproduce these effects in the same strain. The single positive teratogenic study also suffered from an inadequate specification for the dye employed. The committee took account of the fact that the new data, in addition to the new information on the deficiency of the specification of amaranth in the positive studies previously reviewed, allowed for more precise assessment of the ADI.

ADI   0–0.5 mg/kg body weight

Maximum allowable levels
70 mg/L in beverages and 290 mg/kg foods other than beverages

Used in   fruit flavoured drinks, jelly, confectionery, carbonated soft drinks

124   Ponceau 4R or Brilliant scarlet 4R (CI 16255)

Source   Synthesised from coal tar.

Function   Dye or lake dye bright red stable to pH and temperatures of processing and storage.

Properties   According to the World Health Organisation, several long-term studies specifically designed for carcinogenesis only have been performed in the rat, and another 80-week study in the mouse is now available. Teratology has been examined in the mouse and a short-term study in a non-rodent species has been performed. There is little information on the metabolism of this colour.

ADI   0–4 mg/kg body weight

Maximum allowable levels
70 mg/L in beverages and 290 mg/kg foods other than beverages

Used in   cakes, biscuits, frozen desserts, sauces, soft drinks, confectionery, packet sauce mixes

127 Erythrosine or Red 3, (CI45430)

Source Synthesised from the coal tar fluorescein to tetraiodofluorescein, as the disodium salt.

Function Dye or lake dye raspberry red to dark red. Because it is insoluble in acid, it is added to cherries before canning and the pigment remains on the cherries as a precipitate.

Properties Professor Tanaka from Hyakunincho University, Tokyo, fed erythrosine in large amounts to mice from five weeks of age of the F_0 generation to nine weeks of age of the F_1 generation in mice, and selected reproductive and neurobehavioural parameters were measured. There were no adverse effects of erythrosine on either litter size, litter weight or sex ratio at birth. The average body weight of the offspring was significantly increased in the middle-dose group of both sexes during the lactation period. In behavioural developmental parameters, any variables showed no significant adverse effects in either sex in the lactation period. In movement activity of exploratory behaviour, several parameters were significantly changed in the high-dose group, and those effects were dose related in adult females in the F_0 and F_1 generations and in male offspring in the F_1 generation. The dose level of erythrosine in the present study produced few adverse effects in reproductive and neurobehavioural parameters in mice.

ADI 0–0.1 mg/kg body weight

Maximum allowable levels
70 mg/L in beverages and 290 mg/kg foods other than beverages

Used in canned fruit, jams, jelly, cheese rind, cakes, biscuits, soft drinks, confectionery

129   Allura red AC (CI 16035)

Source   Synthesised from coal tar as an azo dye.

Function   Dye or lake red dye.

Properties   Some experiments with test animals have found negative health problems with the use of Allura red but the doses have been at 2 mg/kg yet the ADI is 0–7 mg/kg!

According to the World Health Organisation, a variety of mutagenicity studies carried out with Allura red indicated that there were no mutagenic effects. Another study on acute and short-term oral toxicity of Allura red in several species revealed that apart from the coloration of the urine and faeces, there were no other compound-related responses. Dermal studies (both short- and long-term) also indicated an absence of colour-induced toxic responses. In long-term feeding studies on mice and rats, the most consistent observation was that the animals that received the greatest amount of colour (51.9 g/kg of food) exhibited lower body weights compared to control animals. One study suggested that mice that were fed on this colour demonstrated an earlier onset of tumours of the lymphatic system compared to control mice. However, a second, more extensive mouse study has not borne this out. The long-term study and the mutagenicity studies suggest that Allura red does not possess carcinogenic potential.

ADI   0–7 mg/kg body weight

Maximum allowable levels
70 mg/L in beverages and 290 mg/kg foods other than beverages

Used in   soft drinks, confectionery, cakes, biscuits, sauce mixes, stir-fry mixes

132   Indigotine or indigo carmine or blue 2 (CI 73015)

Source   Manufactured from coal tar or petroleum.

Function   Blue dye or lake dye.

Properties   The World Health Organisation has been concerned about indigotine because the production of a high percentage of local sarcomata at the site of subcutaneous injections in rats led in the past to considerable discussion and consequently to extensive studies on this colour and the special condition of the experiment and does not constitute evidence of carcinogenicity by the oral route. The metabolic studies on this colour are fairly complete and the two long-term studies in the rat do not point to any significant toxic effects. A 13-week study on the major metabolite revealed no toxic effects. Human metabolic studies would be useful.

ADI   0–5 mg/kg body weight

Used in   caviar, baked products, confectionery, ice confections, yoghurt

133   Brilliant blue FCF or blue 2 (CI 42900)

Source   Synthesised from coal tar to disodium sulfonatobenzyl-amino-phenyl-2-sulfonatophenyl-methylene-cyclohexadiene.

Function   Blue dye or lake dye.

Properties   No adverse report. According to the World Health Organisation, "Biochemical studies have shown that the colour is poorly absorbed and is almost completely excreted in the faeces after parenteral administration. Extensive long-term studies in two species are available. In addition, a 13-week study in rats with o-sulfobenzaldehyde, one of the components of commercial Brilliant blue FCF, has been carried out. Oral feeding produced no pathological changes at the highest levels used in adequate experiments."

ADI   0–12.5 mg/kg body weight

Maximum allowable levels
70 mg/L in beverages and 290 mg/kg foods other than beverages

Used in   soft drinks, confectionery, cakes, biscuits, sauce mixes, stir-fry mixes

140   Chlorophyll (CI 758100)

Source   Extracted by solvent from green grass, lucerne and other plant matter to give phaeophytins wholly or partially bound to magnesium salts naturally present in the original plant material. Other pigments such as carotenes may be present.

Function   "Natural" dark green colour.

Properties   Chlorophyll has been a natural part of people's diet and there are no health concerns. The Internet is full of people ringing the praises of chlorophyll drinks and pills as health foods but there is no scientific evidence to support such claims.

ADI   No ADI

Used in   fruit leathers, sauces, green curry pastes, soups, pea puree

141   Chlorophyll-copper complex (CI 75810)

Source   Copper salts (alkaline) are added to extracts obtained by extracting chlorophyll by solvent from green grass, lucerne and other plant matter to replace the magnesium complex with copper phaeophytins salts. Other pigments such as carotenes may be present.

Function Olive green copper complexes that are soluble in vegetable oils.

Properties No adverse effects

ADI 0–15 mg/kg body weight

Used in olive puree, pizza toppings, dips and spreads

142 Green S or acid brilliant green BS or food green S or lissamine green (CI 44090)

Source Derived from the naphthalene coal tar.

Function Green dye or lake dye.

Properties No subcutaneous sarcomata were seen in control rats (24 male and 24 female rats were dosed with distilled water in parallel as controls). The average life-span of the test animals was 21 months and for the control animals 24 months. The average life-span of the test animals was 30 months, the control animals 24 months.

ADI 0–1 mg/kg body weight

Maximum allowable levels
70 mg/L in beverages and 290 mg/kg foods other than beverages

Used in confectionery, frozen ice blocks, soft drinks, jelly

143 Fast green FCF (CI 42053)

Source Derived from the naphthalene coal tar.

Function Green dye or lake dye.

Properties The World Health Series 21 states "A review of the histopathological data from a rat trial indicated that Fast green FCF caused cancer".

A carcinogenicity study was performed from which

it was concluded that inappropriate statistical tests had been performed on some of the data by the testing laboratory. Using appropriate statistical procedures the reviewers concluded that there were no significant differences in tumour incidence between combined control groups and the high-dose group with respect to tumours of the liver, testes or thyroid; the tissues from the low and intermediate-dose groups were not examined. In a blind review of the slides of the bladders from all dose groups, only three proliferative lesions, two benign (papilloma) and one malignant (carcinoma), were observed in bladders of male rats in the high-dose group and a treatment-related increase in the incidence or severity of transitional cell hyperplasia was not detected. It was concluded that the observation of only three neoplasms in the high-dose male group, two of which were of questionable neoplastic character, and the absence of evidence of a pre-neoplastic process in the observed hyperplasia, established that there is no indication of a neoplastic effect on the urinary bladder from administration of Fast green FCF.

ADI   0–5 mg/kg body weight

Maximum allowable levels
          70 mg/L in beverages and 290 mg/kg foods other than beverages

Used in   condiments, dairy foods, syrups, sauces, confectionery

150a   Caramel I

Source   The caramels are different from the "caramel" made by boiling sugar solutions in the kitchen or restaurant. These caramels are black solids or liquids made by controlled heating of invert sugar, sucrose or glucose with sulphur dioxide and/or sodium hydroxide or ammonia or acid. Caramel Colour I (synonyms: plain caramel, caustic caramel, and spirit caramel), this class is prepared by the controlled heat treatment of carbohydrates with alkali or acid.

Function Caramel I imparts a stable brown colour to foods.

Properties According to the World Health Organisation, "Caramel Colour I is free of the heterocyclic compounds associated with convulsant activity or depressed lymphocyte counts which occur in caramels prepared using impure ammonia or ammonium salts, and displays a low order of short-term toxicity. None of the data suggest a need to revise earlier JECFA recommendations."

ADI 0–200 mg/kg body weight

Maximum allowable levels
70 mg/L in beverages and 290 mg/kg foods other than beverages

Used in beer, whisky, brandy, rum, baked goods, confectionery, ginger beer, soft drinks, gravy mixes, sauces

150b Caramel II

Source Caramel Colour II (synonyms: caustic sulphite process caramel), this class is prepared by the controlled heat treatment of carbohydrates with sulphite-containing compounds.

Function Imparts a stable brown colour to foods.

Properties See Caramel I.

ADI No ADI

Maximum allowable levels
70 mg/L in beverages and 290 mg/kg foods other than beverages

Used in	beer, whisky, rum, baked goods, confectionery, ginger beer, soft drinks, gravy mixes, sauces

150c   Caramel III

Source	Caramel Colour III (synonyms: ammonia caramel, ammonia process caramel, closed-pan ammonia process caramel, open-pan ammonia process caramel, bakers' caramel, confectioners' caramel, and beer caramel), this class is prepared by the controlled heat treatment of carbohydrates with ammonium compounds.
Function	Imparts a stable brown colour to foods.
Properties	See Caramel I.
ADI	0–200 mg/kg body weight

Maximum allowable levels

70 mg/L in beverages and 290 mg/kg foods other than beverages

Used in	spreads, soups, beer, whisky, rum, baked goods, confectionery, ginger beer, soft drinks, gravy mixes, sauces

150d   Caramel IV

Source	Caramel Colour IV (synonyms: ammonia sulphite process caramel, sulphite ammonia caramel, sulphite ammonia process caramel, acid-proof caramel, beverage caramel, and soft-drink caramel), this class is prepared by the controlled heat treatment of carbohydrates with ammonium-containing and sulphite-containing compounds.
Function	Imparts a stable brown colour to foods.
Properties	See Caramel I.

ADI   No ADI

Maximum allowable levels
70 mg/L in beverages and 290 mg/kg foods other than beverages

Used in   breakfast cereals, rum, biscuits, cakes, confectionery, ginger beer, soft drinks, gravy mixes, sauces

151   Brilliant black BN or Brilliant black PN

Source   Synthesised from coal tar.

Function   Black dye or lake dye stable in acidic foods.

Properties   Brilliant black PN was non-mutagenic in liquid fluctuation assays using an *E-coli* strain sensitive to base substitutions and a *Salmonella typhimurium* specific for frame shifts. The colour did not produce DNA damage to a repair deficient strain of *E-coli*, with or without microsomal activation.

A multigenerational study was performed on Wistar rats in which the colourant was administered in the diet at concentrations of 0, 0.1, 1.0 or 3% for three successive generations. One litter was reared from each of the F_0, F_1 and F_2 parents. Each generation started with 60 animals of each sex in the control group and 40 of each sex in the test groups. After a nine-week test period, 24 males and 24 females from the control group, and 14 males and 14 females from each test group were used for teratogenicity studies; the remainder were used for the reproduction study. No adverse effects were observed with respect to fertility, litter size and weight, general condition, male/female ratio, growth during lactation, survival or maturation. Autopsy of parent rats and pups at weaning did not reveal any treatment related changes in organ weights other than caecal enlargement in the 3% dose group. Gross and microscopic examination of the F3 generation at weaning did not reveal any abnormalities due to treatment and no adverse effects were seen in the teratology study. It was concluded that Brilliant black PN did not exert any adverse effects on reproductive function of Wistar rats when fed at dietary levels up to 3% (1500 mg/kg body weight per day) for three successive generations.

ADI   0–1 mg/kg body weight

Maximum allowable levels
70 mg/L in beverages and 290 mg/kg foods other than beverages

Used in   stout, gravies, soft drinks, confectionery

153   Carbon black or vegetable carbon

Source   Carbon black (vegetable carbon) is derived from partial combustion of vegetable material in furnaces with small amounts of oxygen only to prevent the loss of carbon to carbon dioxide and is produced as a fine powder to form insoluble carbon.

Function   Carbon black is a very stable to processing temperatures, storage and oxidation and provides light black-grey to black hue. Carbon black is not insoluble in water but water-dispersible suspensions have been developed for a range of applications. The main application areas as part of a blend with other colours (such as red and brown pigments) to provide chocolate brown shades.

Properties   Carbon black adsorbs toxins in the gastrointestinal system. According to the World Health Organisation, the available ingestion studies referred only to mice and produced no evidence that activated vegetable carbon exerted any adverse biological effects in this species.

ADI   No ADI

Maximum allowable levels

> 70 mg/L in beverages and 290 mg/kg foods other than beverages

Used in   baked goods, sauces, confectionery, ice cream, compound chocolate

155   Brown HT

Source   Synthesised from coal tar.

Function   Dark brown dye, with the colour of chocolate.

Properties   The World Health Organisation carried out experiments with brown HT. Groups of 48 male and 48 female rats (Wistar strain) were given diets containing 0 (control), 500, 2,000 or 10,000 ppm Chocolate Brown HT (purity minimal 85%) for two years. These treatments had no adverse effect on the bodyweight gain, food or water consumption, haematology, renal function, serum constituents and organ weights. The mortality was only slightly increased in the males with the highest dose level of the dye. The results of the histopathological examination showed no adverse effects except that in the mammary glands a non-significant ("dose-related") increase of the occurrence of fibroadenosis was seen. The incidence of tumours in the treated animals was not different from the control animals

ADI   0–1.5 mg/kg body weight

Maximum allowable levels

> 70 mg/L in beverages and 290 mg/kg foods other than beverages

Used in   baked goods, artificial (compound) chocolate, confectionery

160   β-Carotene

Source   Organic solvent extract of coloured algae and higher plants such as carrots. The carotenes are brightly coloured yellow and orange pigments that are soluble in oil and are found in oranges, peaches, apricots, carrots and dark green vegetables such as broccoli. After consumption, carotenes are absorbed in the small intestine and then transported to the liver. Here they are converted into vitamin A, the vitamin responsible for colour and contrast vision and synthesis of mucopolysaccharides that protect the lungs and gastrointestinal tract.

Function   Yellow and orange pigments that are soluble in oil but not in water. The pigments are destroyed by sunlight but are stable to processing and pH changes. Sulphur dioxide stabilises the carotenes.

Properties   Six grams of carotene can be converted in the body to one gram of vitamin A. Recent research shows that carotene protects the lungs from the harmful effects of smoking and air pollution. Because it is a natural compound, it is replacing some of the yellow coal tar dyes (quinoline yellow, sunset yellow and tartrazine) in processed foods.

ADI   0–5 mg/kg

Group ADI expressed as the sum of the carotenoids: β-carotene, β-apo-8'-carotenal and β-apo-8'-carotenoic acid, methyl and ethyl esters.

Maximum allowable levels

70 mg/L in beverages and 290 mg/kg foods other than beverages

Used in   margarine, dips, pâté, ice cream, confectionery

160b   Annatto extracts (*Bixa orellana L*)

Source
Brazil in South America is the main producer and exporter. Today annatto is also grown in the Philippines as it was introduced by the Spanish.

The red colour comes from many apocarotenoids found in the skin of the seed, of which bixin (9'Z-6, 6'-diapocarotene-6, 6'-dioate) is the most abundant. Other carotenoids and apocarotenoids have been found and their total concentration varies, but may reach up to 8% of the dry seed mass.

Function
The food industry makes use of annatto food colour in the form of various liquid and powder extracts which provide a range of hues from natural banana hue to cherry red. Annatto is stable in foods during storage and does not react with other food additives.

Properties
Oil soluble yellow-coloured dye which is used to give butter, cheese and foods a natural yellow colour.

ADI
0–0.065 mg/kg body weight

Maximum allowable levels
70 mg/L in beverages and 290 mg/kg foods other than beverages

Used in
packaged cake mixes, cheese, margarine, liquorice, dips

160c   Paprika oleoresins

Source
Organic solvents are used to extract the colour components of paprika.

Function
Used as a fat-soluble natural food colour. To mix it into aqueous foods it is adsorbed onto a dry carrier such as salt or maltodextrin.

Properties
There is much interest in the role of dietary carotenoids in the prevention of degenerative

diseases such as cancer and cardiovascular disease. Epidemiological studies suggest that the incidence of human cancer is inversely correlated with the dietary intake of carotenoids and their concentration in blood plasma. However, there have been contradictory reports concerning the use of β-carotene for cancer prevention. It has been demonstrated recently that supplementation of β-carotene in healthy men produced neither benefit nor harm in terms of the incidence of cancer and cardiovascular disease.

ADI   No ADI

Used in   Mexican foods and spices, marinades, sauces, laying-bird rations to add colour to egg yolk

160d   Lycopene

Source   A bright red carotenoid pigment (phytochemical) found in tomatoes and other red fruits. Lycopene is the most common carotenoid in the human body and is one of the most potent carotenoid antioxidants. Its name is derived from the tomato's species classification, *Solanum lycopersicum*. The highest natural concentrations of lycopene in food are found not in tomatoes, but in watermelon. Almost all dietary lycopene comes from tomato products.

Function   Imparts a red colour to foods.

Properties Research has shown that lycopene may prevent prostate, lung and stomach cancer. Lycopene is more bioavailable from processed foods such as tomato juice and tomato sauce than from fruit.

ADI   No ADI

Used in   health bars, sauces, taco mixes

160e β-apo-8' Carotenal

Source   Synthetic forms of the natural substance are used.

Function   Yellow/ red pigment.

Properties Acts like other carotenoids as an antioxidant with potential health benefits.

ADI   0–5 mg/kg body weight

Group ADI expressed as the sum of the carotenoids: β-carotene, β-apo-8'-carotenal and β-apo-8'-carotenoic acid, methyl and ethyl esters.

Used in   cheese dips, pâté, corn chips, burrito mixes

160f β-apo-8' Carotenoic acid or methyl ethyl ester

Source   Synthetic forms of the natural substance are used.

Function   Orange/red pigment.

Properties Acts like other carotenoids as an antioxidant with potential health benefits.

ADI   0–5 mg/kg body weight

Group ADI expressed as the sum of the carotenoids: β-carotene, β-apo-8'-carotenal and β-apo-8'-carotenoic acid, methyl and ethyl esters.

Used in   cheese dips, Mexican foods, liquorice, soup mixes

161a Flavoxanthin (one of the Xanthophylls)

Source   Occurs naturally in many plants and is commercially extracted from buttercup (*Ranunculus* species).

Function   Used as a natural yellow colouring in food. Sparingly soluble in water.

Properties Acts like other carotenoids as an antioxidant with potential health benefits.

ADI   No ADI

Used in   curry powders, savoury spreads, Mexican foods, soups, sauces

161b   Lutein (one of the Xanthophylls)

Source   A yellow pigment in the chemical family of carotenoids and found in egg yolks, vegetables, marigold flowers, alfalfa and to a lesser degree in many other plants.

Function   Used as an intense natural yellow colour in foods. Soluble in water.

Properties   Research has shown that the lutein protects against cataracts and macular degeneration, two most common age-related eye disorders. Lutein is found in the retina and absorbs ultraviolet light that can harm the eye. It has been shown that lutein protects against the blocking of the arteries in the neck and heart muscle. The study, at the University of Southern California, found that participants with the highest levels of lutein in the blood at the outset had no increase in plaque in the arteries throughout the two-year study. There was no effect with the control diet. Dr Landrum from Florida International University has found that evidence both in the laboratory and in human subjects has linked lutein in the diet to the protection of the retina from the risk of getting the debilitating disease; age-related macular degeneration. Lutein also protects against cataracts in the eye.

ADI   No ADI

Used in   health powders and drinks, health bars, baked products

161c Kryptoxanthin, Cryptoxanthin (one of the Xanthophylls)

Source Extracted from the *Solanaceae* Bladder cherry or as a synthetic form.

Function Yellow pigment.

Properties Acts like other carotenoids as an antioxidant with potential health benefits. Dr Landrum from Florida International University has found that evidence both in the laboratory and in human subjects has linked Kryptoxanthin and lutein in the diet to the protection of the retina from the risk of getting the debilitating disease; age-related macular degeneration. This is the leading cause of blindness in individuals over 55 years of age. Research has shown a 43% reduction the risk of cataract has also been shown with high intakes of Kryptoxanthin.

ADI No ADI

Used in cosmetics

161d Rubixanthin (one of the Xanthophylls)

Source Found in the skins of the fruit of many plants. Synthesised commercially (nature identical).

Function Yellow pigment.

Properties Acts like other carotenoids as an antioxidant with potential health benefits.

ADI No ADI

Used in cosmetics

161e Violoxanthin (one of the Xanthophylls)

Source Found in the skins of the fruit of many plants. Synthesised commercially (nature identical).

Function Yellow pigment.

Properties Acts like other carotenoids as an antioxidant with potential health benefits. No toxic properties.

ADI No ADI

Used in cosmetics

161f Rhodoxanthin (one of the Xanthophylls)

Source Found in the skins of the fruit of many plants. Synthesised commercially (nature identical).

Function Yellow food colour, sparingly soluble in water.

Properties Acts like other carotenoids as an antioxidant with potential health benefits.

ADI No ADI

Used in cosmetics, confectionery, vegan foods

162 Beet red (Betanin)

Source Beet red is extracted from beetroot by hot aqueous acid solutions.

Function Beet red is water soluble and is unstable to ultraviolet light, oxygen and high temperatures of processing and prolonged storage.

Properties No adverse effects at levels used in foods. Beet red is an antioxidant that protects the lining of blood vessels from damage.

ADI No ADI

Used in frozen, dried and short shelf-life products (ice creams and yoghurt)

163 Anthocyanins or grape skin extract or blackcurrant extract

Source   Extracted from the skins of grapes after pressing the juice. The extract is dried and may contain tannins and antioxidants.

Function   Bright blue, violet or red pigment with associated antioxidants and grape tannins. The pH of the food controls the colour (red in high acid foods and blue in low acid foods). Anthocyanin pigments found in grape skin extract are made up of diglucosides, monoglucosides, acylated monoglucosides, and acylated diglucosides of peonidin, malvidin, cyanidin, petunidin and delphinidin. The concentration of each compound varies depending upon the grape variety, soil type and climatic conditions.

Tannins that may also be present are monomers or polymers and give beverages a pleasant astringent taste, while the particular antioxidants (cis- and trans-resveratrol) are the most powerful ones in the plant kingdom.

Properties   Antioxidant properties have been researched and found to be protective of blood vessel walls.

ADI   No ADI

Used in   wine, cocktails, soft drinks, health bars

164 Saffron or crocetin or crocin

Source   Saffron is the most expensive spice in the world. The saffron threads are the sun-dried stigmas of the saffron flower, *Crocus Sativus Linneaus*. There are three stigmas in each flower. The stigmas are picked from each flower by hand, and more than 120,000 of these flowers are needed to produce just one kilogram. Saffron is worth more than gold on a weight basis! Other forms of the pigment such as crocetin or crocin are found in the filaments of the fruit of *Gardenia jasminoides Ellis*, a native of China where it is used as a medicine and clothing dye.

Function   Yellow, slightly bitter powder or threads which are soluble in water and alcohol.

Properties   Saffron has hormone-like effects and the anti-carcinogenic and anti-toxic effects have been measured in humans. Saffron has also been used to treat arthrosclerosis and arthritis.

ADI   No ADI

Used in   Because of the expense it is used in high class restaurants to flavour rice and various sauces.

170   Calcium carbonate (CI 77220)

Source   Obtained from natural deposits of limestone. Analyses must be carried out to determine the heavy metal (lead, mercury and cadmium) content.

Function   White opaque pigment and anti-caking agent because it absorbs moisture readily.

Properties   No adverse effects and calcium carbonate adds calcium to the diet.

ADI   No ADI

Used in   cake mixes, baked goods, confectionery, canned vegetables

171   Titanium dioxide (CI 77891)

Source   Titanium dioxide is refined from underground ore deposits and it exists in a number of crystalline forms as ilmenite or leuxocene in found as lumps of rutile in beach sand. Also known as the mineral ilmenite, (named after the Ilmen Mountains in Russia).

Function	Opaque pigment, insoluble in water and alcohol. It is used in food as well as in packaging to protect foods from ultraviolet light.
Properties	No adverse health affects as it is not to be easily absorbed, although detectable amounts can be found in the blood, brain and glands with the highest concentrations being in the lymph nodes and lungs. It is excreted from the body with urine.
ADI	No ADI but 5 g/kg allowed in Australian foods
Used in	confectionery, cake decorating

172   Iron oxide (CI 77492, yellow or 77491 red or 77499, black)

Source	Naturally occurring oxides of iron with red, yellow or black colours.
Function	Insoluble pigments in foods.
Properties	According to the World Health Organisation Expert Committee on Food Additives, "Iron oxides are permitted for use in foods in the draft General Standard for Food Additives being established by the Codex Committee on Food Additives and Contaminants, the use being limited only by good manufacturing practice. The Committee assessed national estimates of intake of iron oxides used as additives for colouring food. Use of iron oxides is permitted in most countries. Data were submitted by four countries: Australia, Canada, the United Kingdom, and the US. Current use of iron oxides as a food colour is very limited, and the intakes based on national standards do not exceed the ADI. The Committee concluded that it is unlikely that the intake of iron oxides will exceed the ADI."
ADI	0–0.5 mg/kg body weight
Used in	sausage casing, pâté

173   Aluminium (CI 77000)

Source   Extracted by electrolysis from the natural bauxite ore.

Function   Used as an insoluble carrier of opaque food dyes.

Properties   There is an increasing body of published research that suggests that an accumulation of aluminium in the cells of the brain and other nerve tissues is toxic. It is present in abnormally high levels in the form of organic aluminium in the brain cells of Alzheimer's disease sufferers, accumulated in the neurofibrillary tangles and neuritic plaques. It is not known whether this is a "cause and effect", resulting in the disease.

Several reports also suggest that a high aluminium intake may have adverse effects on the metabolism of phosphorous and calcium in the human body and may induce or intensify skeletal abnormalities such as osteoporosis.

ADI   0–0.5 mg/kg body weight

Used in   food packaging, confectionery

174   Silver (CI 77820)

Source   Produced from electrolysis of silver ore using the Thum Balbach or Moebius patent methods.

Function   As a food additive it is used solely for external decoration where it can be found on chocolate confectionery, in the covering of dragées and the decoration of sugar-coated flour confectionery

Properties   Prolonged, regular consumption can lead to grey discoloration of the eyes and kidney damage, nasal and nose septum, throat and skin.

ADI   No ADI

Used in   specialised confectionery, Indian cuisine

175   Gold (CI 77480)

Source   Occurs in the pure form as it does not react with any other compound.

Function   Small, thin leaves are used in exotic foods.

Properties   Completely inert and passes through the gastrointestinal tract unchanged.

ADI   No ADI

Used in   Indian cuisine, confectionery, liqueurs

181   Tannic acid or tannins: Gallotannin or Gallotannic acid or Digallic Acid or Glycerite or Tannin

Source   Extracted from galls of chestnuts, seed pods of the Tara plant. Also extracted from oak, in particular, wine is aged in oak barrels and the natural oak tannin dissolves in the wine.

Function   Colour, emulsifier, stabiliser, thickener, taste modulating, clarifying and refining agent in beverages.

Properties   No adverse effects

ADI   No ADI

Used in   beer (12 mg/L, permitted), wine (12 mg/L, permitted), wine coolers (12 mg/L, permitted)

200 PRESERVATIVES AND FOOD ACIDS

200   Sorbic acid

Source   Sorbic acid is a white, crystalline solid synthesised from oil. It has a mildly acrid odour.

Function   Antimicrobial and fungistatic agent. Sorbic acid is particularly effective against surface moulds. In wine it can sometimes be metabolised by bacteria to a compound that gives the wine the flavour of geraniums. Sorbic acid is effective at higher pH (6.5) than other preservatives such as the benzoates.

Properties   No adverse effects at levels used in foods.

ADI   0–25 mg/kg body weight (take into account the sum of additives 200–203

Used in   fresh fruit salad (375 mg/kg), dips (500 mg/kg), fruit drinks (400 mg/kg), fruit juice drinks (400 mg/kg), fruit juices (400 mg/kg), fruit flavoured drinks (400 mg/kg), flour (1,000 mg/kg), cheese (3,000 mg/kg), ginger beer (400 mg/kg), bread (1.2 g/kg), cider (400 mg/kg), wine (200 mg/kg), liquorice (1 g/kg), olives in brine (400 mg/kg), reduced fat cheese and spreads (3 g/kg), cheese slices (2 g/kg), tomato juice (400 mg/kg)

201   Sodium sorbate

Source   Manufactured by adding caustic soda to sorbic acid.

Function   Preservative.

Properties   No adverse effects

ADI   0–25 mg/kg body weight

Used in   The ANZFS code suggests that a good manufacturing practice is to use no more than 500 mg/kg food.

fresh fruit salad (375 mg/kg), dips (500 mg/kg), fruit drinks (400 mg/kg), fruit juice drinks (400 mg/kg), fruit juices (400 mg/kg), fruit flavoured drinks (400 mg/kg), flour (1,000 mg/kg), cheese (3,000 mg/kg), ginger beer (400 mg/kg), bread (1.2 g/kg), cider (400 mg/kg), wine (200 mg/kg), liquorice (1 g/kg), olives in brine (400 mg/kg), reduced fat cheese and spreads (3 g/kg), cheese slices (2 g/kg), tomato juice (400 mg/kg)

202   Potassium sorbate

Source   Manufactured by adding potassium hydroxide to sorbic acid.

Function   Anti-mould and anti-bacterial agent.

Properties No adverse effects

ADI   0–25 mg/kg body weight

Used in   The ANZFS code suggests that a good manufacturing practice is to use no more than 1,000 g/kg food.

fresh fruit salad (375 mg/kg), dips (500 mg/kg), fruit drinks (400 mg/kg), fruit juice drinks (400 mg/kg), fruit juices (400 mg/kg), fruit flavoured drinks (400 mg/kg), flour (1,000 mg/kg), cheese (3,000 mg/kg), ginger beer (400 mg/kg), bread (1.2 g/kg), cider (400 mg/kg), wine (200 mg/kg), liquorice (1 g/kg), olives in brine (400 mg/kg), reduced fat cheese and spreads (3 g/kg), cheese slices (2 g/kg), tomato juice (400 mg/kg)

203   Calcium sorbate

Source   Manufactured by adding lime to sorbic acid.

Function   Anti-mould (surface of food) and anti-bacterial.

Properties No adverse effects

ADI   0–25mg/kg body weight

Used in   The ANZFS code suggests that a good manufacturing practice is to use no more than 500 mg/kg food.

fresh fruit salad (375 mg/kg), dips (500 mg/kg), fruit drinks (400 mg/kg), fruit juice drinks (400 mg/kg), fruit juices (400 mg/kg), fruit flavoured drinks (400 mg/kg), flour (1,000 mg/kg), cheese (3,000 mg/kg), ginger beer (400 mg/kg), bread (1.2 g/kg), cider (400 mg/kg), wine (200 mg/kg), liquorice (1 g/kg), olives in brine (400 mg/kg), reduced fat cheese and spreads (3 g/kg), cheese slices (2 g/kg), tomato juice (400 mg/kg)

210   Benzoic acid or carboxy benzene

Source   Synthesised from petroleum fraction benzene, sulphuric acid followed by carbon dioxide addition.

Function   Not very soluble in beverages. Anti-mould and anti-bacterial agent. Only effective in acid foods (pH < 5.5) as the undissociated molecule is the effective molecule. Benzoic acid acts synergistically with sorbic acid and sulphur dioxide.

Properties   There have been controversial findings about benzoic acid and health because of its chemical similarities to salicylate. Some studies have suggested that benzoic acid can aggravate attention disorders, asthma and dermatitis while others have found no adverse reactions in humans given 1,000 times the ADI! The kidneys metabolise and remove benzoic acid in less than 16 hours.

ADI   0–25 mg/kg body weight

Used in   The ANZFS code suggests that a good manufacturing practice is to use no more than 500 mg/kg food.

fresh fruit salad (375 mg/kg), dips (500 mg/kg), fruit drinks (400 mg/kg), fruit juice drinks (400 mg/kg), fruit juices (400 mg/kg), fruit flavoured drinks (400 mg/kg), flour (1,000 mg/kg), cheese (3,000 mg/kg), ginger beer (400 mg/kg), bread (1.2 g/kg), cider (400 mg/kg), wine (200 mg/kg), liquorice (1 g/kg), olives in brine (400 mg/kg), reduced fat cheese and spreads (3 g/kg), cheese slices (2 g/kg), tomato juice (400 mg/kg), low-joule jams (1g/kg), cordial (800 mg/kg)

211   Sodium benzoate

Source   Synthesised by adding caustic soda to benzoic acid.

Function   More soluble in beverages than benzoic acid. Anti-mould and anti-bacterial agent. Only effective in acid foods (pH < 5.5) as the undissociated molecule is the effective molecule. Benzoic acid acts synergistically with sorbic acid and sulphur dioxide.

Properties There have been controversial findings about benzoic acid and health because of its chemical similarities to salicylate. Some studies have suggested that benzoic acid can aggravate attention disorders, asthma and dermatitis while others have found no adverse reactions in humans given 1,000 times the ADI! The kidneys metabolise and remove benzoic acid in less than 16 hours.

ADI   0–25 mg/kg body weight

Used in   The ANZFS code suggests that a good manufacturing practice is to use no more than 500 mg/kg food.

fresh fruit salad (375 mg/kg), dips (500 mg/kg), fruit drinks (400 mg/kg), fruit juice drinks (400 mg/kg), fruit juices (400 mg/kg), fruit flavoured drinks (400 mg/kg), flour (1,000 mg/kg), cheese (3,000 mg/kg), ginger beer (400 mg/kg), bread (1.2 g/kg), cider (400 mg/kg), wine (200 mg/kg), liquorice (1 g/kg), olives in brine (400 mg/kg), reduced fat cheese and spreads (3 g/kg), cheese slices (2 g/kg), tomato juice (400 mg/kg), low-joule jams (1g/kg), cordial (800 mg/kg)

212 Potassium benzoate

Source Manufactured by treating aqueous solution of benzoic acid with potassium hydroxide.

Function Anti-mould and anti-bacterial agent. Only effective in acid foods (pH < 5.5) as the undissociated molecule is the effective molecule. Benzoic acid acts synergistically with sorbic acid and sulphur dioxide.

Properties There have been controversial findings about benzoic acid and health because of its chemical similarities to salicylate. Some studies have suggested that benzoic acid can aggravate attention disorders, asthma and dermatitis while others have found no adverse reactions in humans given 1,000 times the ADI! The kidneys metabolise and remove benzoic acid in less than 16 hours.

ADI 0–25 mg/kg body weight

Used in The ANZFS code suggests that a good manufacturing practice is to use no more than 500 mg/kg food.

fresh fruit salad (375 mg/kg), dips (500 mg/kg), fruit drinks (400 mg/kg), fruit juice drinks (400 mg/kg), fruit juices (400 mg/kg), fruit flavoured drinks (400 mg/kg), flour (1,000 mg/kg), cheese (3,000 mg/kg), ginger beer (400 mg/kg), bread (1.2 g/kg), cider (400 mg/kg), wine (200 mg/kg), liquorice (1 g/kg), olives in brine (400 mg/kg), reduced fat cheese and spreads (3 g/kg), cheese slices (2 g/kg), tomato juice (400 mg/kg), low-joule jam (1 g/kg), cordial (800 mg/kg)

213 Calcium benzoate

Source Manufactured by treating an aqueous solution of benzoic acid with lime (calcium hydroxide).

Function Anti-mould and anti-bacterial agent. Only effective in acid foods (pH < 5.5) as the undissociated molecule is the effective molecule. Benzoic acid acts synergistically with sorbic acid and sulphur dioxide.

Properties There have been controversial findings about benzoic acid and health because of its chemical similarities to salicylate. Some studies have suggested that benzoic acid can aggravate attention disorders, asthma and dermatitis while others have found no adverse reactions in humans given 1,000 times the ADI! The kidneys metabolise and remove benzoic acid in less than 16 hours.

ADI 0–25 mg/kg body weight

Used in The ANZFS code suggests that a good manufacturing practice is to use no more than 500 mg/kg food.

fresh fruit salad (375 mg/kg), dips (500 mg/kg), fruit drinks (400 mg/kg), fruit juice drinks (400 mg/kg), fruit juices (400 mg/kg), fruit flavoured drinks (400 mg/kg), flour (1,000 mg/kg), cheese (3,000 mg/kg), ginger beer (400 mg/kg), bread (1.2 g/kg), cider (400 mg/kg), wine (200 mg/kg), liquorice (1 g/kg), olives in brine (400 mg/kg), reduced fat cheese and spreads (3 g/kg), cheese slices (2 g/kg), tomato juice (400 mg/kg), low-joule jams (1 g/kg), cordial (800 mg/kg)

216   Propylparaben or Propyl-p-hydroxy-benzoate

Source Synthesised by propylation and hydroxylation of benzoic acid.

Function More soluble in foods than benzoic acid. Effective over a wider pH than benzoic acid. Anti-mould and anti-bacterial agent. Only effective in acid foods (pH < 6.5) as the undissociated molecule is the effective molecule. Benzoic acid acts synergistically with sorbic acid and sulphur dioxide.

Properties There have been controversial findings about benzoic acid and health because of its chemical similarities to salicylate. Some studies have suggested that benzoic acid can aggravate attention disorders, asthma and dermatitis while others have found no adverse reactions in humans given 1,000 times the ADI! The kidneys metabolise and remove benzoic acid in less than 16 hours.

ADI   0–25 mg/kg body weight

Used in The ANZFS code suggests that a good manufacturing practice is to use no more than 500 mg/kg food.

fresh fruit salad (375 mg/kg), dips (500 mg/kg), fruit drinks (400 mg/kg), fruit juice drinks (400 mg/kg), fruit juices (400 mg/kg), fruit flavoured drinks (400 mg/kg), flour (1,000 mg/kg), cheese (3,000 mg/kg), ginger beer (400 mg/kg), bread (1.2 g/kg), cider (400 mg/kg), wine (200 mg/kg), liquorice (1 g/kg)olives in brine (400 mg/kg), reduced fat cheese and spreads (3 g/kg), cheese slices (2 g/kg), tomato juice (400 mg/kg), low-joule jams (1 g/kg), cordial (800 mg/kg)

218   Methylparaben or Methyl-p-hydroxy-benzoate

Source   Synthesised by methylation and hydroxylation of benzoic acid.

Function More soluble in water than benzoic acid. Anti-mould and anti-bacterial agent. Effective in acid foods over a wider pH than benzoic acid (pH < 5.5) as the undissociated molecule is the effective molecule. Benzoic acid acts synergistically with sorbic acid and sulphur dioxide.

Properties There have been controversial findings about benzoic acid and health because of its chemical similarities to salicylate. Some studies have suggested that benzoic acid can aggravate attention disorders, asthma and dermatitis while others have found no adverse reactions in humans given 1,000 times the ADI! The kidneys metabolise and remove benzoic acid in less than 16 hours.

ADI   0–25 mg/kg body weight

Used in   The ANZFS code suggests that a good manufacturing practice is to use no more than 500 mg/kg food.

fresh fruit salad (375 mg/kg), dips (500 mg/kg), fruit drinks (400 mg/kg), fruit juice drinks (400 mg/kg), fruit juices (400 mg/kg), fruit flavoured drinks (400 mg/kg), flour (1,000 mg/kg), cheese (3,000 mg/kg), ginger beer (400 mg/kg), bread (1.2 g/kg), cider (400 mg/kg), wine (200 mg/kg), liquorice (1 g/kg), olives in brine (400 mg/kg), reduced fat cheese and spreads (3 g/kg), cheese slices (2 g/kg), tomato juice (400 mg/kg), low-joule jams (1 g/kg), cordial (800 mg/kg)

220   Sulphur dioxide

Source   Manufactured by burning sulphur.

Function   Water soluble gas used as an antioxidant, anti-fungal and anti-bacterial agent and antioxidant. Sulphur dioxide prevents both enzymic browning in fruit and vegetables and non-enzymic browning during processing of foods such as cooking meat or baking bread, biscuits and cakes. Sulphur dioxide prevents ascorbic acid (vitamin C) from being destroyed in fruit and fruit juice. However, sulphur dioxide destroys thiamine (vitamin B1). It is interesting that wine yeast synthesises up to 25 mg/L of sulphur dioxide and "organic wines" are allowed to be made with sulphur dioxide.

Properties I have found that cooking with wine that contains sulphur dioxide removes all of the thiamine from the food. I would suggest that sulphur dioxide should not be allowed in sausages as this product is a source of thiamine.

Sulphur dioxide has been implicated in initiating an asthma attack. Beverages such as wine have been blamed on asthma attacks. However, double blind clinical trials have recently been carried out by Professor Vally in Western Australia and asthmatics intolerant to wine seem to have diminished histamine degradation probably based on a deficiency of diamine oxidase. Acetaldehyde and amines such as histamine seem to be the cause of the attacks.

ADI   0–0.7 mg/kg body weight

Used in   The ANZFS code suggests that a good manufacturing practice is to use no more than 350 mg/kg food. In many cases manufacturers use far less than the recommended levels and sulphur dioxide and sulphites are destroyed rapidly by reducing sugars. For example, wine makers generally use only 50 parts per million of sulphur dioxide or sulphites in the initial stages of fermentation.

beer (25 mg/L), ginger beer (115 mg/L), canned fish (30 mg/kg), cider (200 mg/L), cheese (300 mg/kg), crystallised fruit (280 mg/kg), dried fruit (3 g/kg), dehydrated beans (750 mg/kg), dehydrated peas (200 mg/kg), dehydrated potatoes (500 mg/kg), flavoured cordials (230 mg/L), fruit drinks (115 mg/L), fruit juices (115 mg/L), fruit juice drinks (115 mg/L), gelatine (750 mg/kg), low-joule jams (285 mg/kg), pickles (750 mg/kg), soft drinks (115 mg/kg), sausages, raw (500 mg/kg), tomato juice (115 mg/L), vinegar (100 mg/L), wine (300 mg/L)

221   Sodium sulphite

Source   Manufactured by bubbling sulphur dioxide through a caustic soda solution.

Function   Sodium sulphite has only 51% of the potency of sulphur dioxide. Dry, corrosive powder. Anti-fungal and anti-bacterial agent and antioxidant. Sulphites prevent both enzymic browning in fruit and vegetables and non-enzymic browning during processing of foods such as cooking meat or baking bread, biscuits and cakes. Sulphites prevent ascorbic acid (vitamin C) from being destroyed in fruit and fruit juice. However, sulphites destroy thiamine (vitamin B1).

Properties I have found that cooking with wine that contains sulphites removes all of the thiamine from the food. I would suggest that sulphur dioxide should not be allowed in sausages as this product is a source of thiamine.

Sulphites have been implicated in initiating an asthma attack. Beverages such as wine have been blamed on asthma attacks. However, double blind clinical trials have recently been carried out by Professor Vally in Western Australia and asthmatics intolerant to wine seem to have diminished histamine degradation probably based on a deficiency of diamine oxidase. Acetaldehyde and amines such as histamine seem to be the cause of the attacks.

ADI 0–0.7 mg/kg body weight

Used in The ANZFS code suggests that a good manufacturing practice is to use no more than 350 mg/kg food.

In many cases manufacturers use far less than the recommended levels and sulphur dioxide and sulphites are destroyed rapidly by reducing sugars. For example, wine makers generally use only 50 parts per million of sulphur dioxide or sulphites in the initial stages of fermentation.

beer (25 mg/L), ginger beer (115 mg/L), canned fish (30 mg/kg), cider (200 mg/L), cheese (300 mg/kg), crystallised fruit (280 mg/kg), dried fruit (3 g/kg), dehydrated beans (750 mg/kg), dehydrated peas (200 mg/kg), dehydrated potatoes (500 mg/kg), flavoured cordials (230 mg/L), fruit drinks (115 mg/L), fruit juices (115 mg/L), fruit juice drinks (115 mg/L), gelatine (750 mg/kg), low-joule jams (285 mg/kg), pickles (750 mg/kg), soft drinks (115 mg/kg), sausages, raw (500 mg/kg), tomato juice (115 mg/L), vinegar (100 mg/L), wine (300 mg/L)

222 Sodium bisulphite

Source Manufactured from gaseous sulphur dioxide.

Function Sodium bisulphite has only 75% of the potency of sulphur dioxide. Dry, corrosive powder. Anti-fungal and anti-bacterial agent and antioxidant. Sulphites prevent both enzymic browning in fruit and vegetables and non-enzymic browning during processing of foods such as cooking meat or baking bread, biscuits and cakes. Sulphites prevent ascorbic acid (vitamin C) from being destroyed in fruit and fruit juice. However, sulphites destroy thiamine (vitamin B1).

Properties I have found that cooking with wine that contains sulphur dioxide removes all of the thiamine from the food. I would suggest that sulphur dioxide should not be allowed in sausages as this product is a source of thiamine.

Sulphur dioxide has been implicated in initiating an asthma attack. Beverages such as wine have been blamed on asthma attacks. However, double blind clinical trials have recently been carried out by Professor Vally in Western Australia and asthmatics intolerant to wine seem to have diminished histamine degradation probably based on a deficiency of diamine oxidase. Acetaldehyde and amines such as histamine seem to be the cause of the attacks.

ADI 0–0.7 mg/kg body weight

Used in In many cases manufacturers use far less than the recommended levels and sulphur dioxide and sulphites are destroyed rapidly by reducing sugars. For example, wine makers generally use only 50 parts per million of sulphur dioxide or sulphites in the initial stages of fermentation.

The ANZFS code suggests that a good manufacturing practice is to use no more than 350 mg/kg food.

beer (25 mg/L), ginger beer (115 mg/L), canned fish (30 mg/kg), cider (200 mg/L), cheese (300 mg/kg), crystallised fruit (280 mg/kg), dried fruit (3 g/kg), dehydrated beans (750 mg/kg), dehydrated peas (200 mg/kg), dehydrated potatoes (500 mg/kg), flavoured cordials (230 mg/L), fruit drinks (115 mg/L), fruit juices (115 mg/L), fruit juice drinks (115 mg/L), gelatine (750 mg/kg), low-joule jam (285 mg/kg), pickles (750 mg/kg), soft drinks (115 mg/L), sausages, raw (500 mg/kg), tomato juice (115 mg/L), vinegar (100 mg/L), wine (300 mg/L)

223 Sodium metabisulphite

Source Manufactured from gaseous sulphur dioxide.

Function Sodium metabisulphite has only 67% of the potency of sulphur dioxide. Dry, corrosive powder. Anti-fungal and anti-bacterial agent and antioxidant. Sulphites prevent both enzymic browning in fruit and vegetables and non-enzymic browning during processing of foods such as cooking meat or baking bread, biscuits and cakes. Sulphites prevent ascorbic acid (vitamin C) from being destroyed in fruit and fruit juice. However, sulphites destroy thiamine (vitamin B1).

Properties I have found that cooking with wine that contains sulphur dioxide, removes all of the thiamine from the food. I would suggest that sulphur dioxide should not be allowed in sausages as this product is a source of thiamine.

Sulphur dioxide has been implicated in initiating an asthma attack. Beverages such as wine have been blamed on asthma attacks. However, double blind clinical trials have recently been carried out by Professor Vally in Western Australia and asthmatics intolerant to wine seem to have diminished histamine degradation probably based on a deficiency of diamine oxidase. Acetaldehyde and amines such as histamine seem to be the cause of the attacks.

ADI   0–0.7 mg/kg body weight

Used in   The ANZFS code suggests that a good manufacturing practice is to use no more than 350 mg/kg food.

In many cases manufacturers use far less than the recommended levels and sulphur dioxide and sulphites are destroyed rapidly by reducing sugars. For example, wine makers generally use only 50 parts per million of sulphur dioxide or sulphites in the initial stages of fermentation.

beer (25 mg/L), ginger beer (115 mg/L), canned fish (30 mg/kg), cider (200 mg/L), cheese (300 mg/kg), crystallised fruit (280 mg/kg), dried fruit (3 g/kg), dehydrated beans (750 mg/kg), dehydrated peas (200 mg/kg), dehydrated potatoes (500 mg/kg), flavoured cordials (230 mg/L), fruit drinks (115 mg/L), fruit juices (115 mg/L), fruit juice drinks (115 mg/L), gelatine (750 mg/kg), low-joule jam (285 mg/kg), pickles (750 mg/kg), soft drinks (115 mg/L), sausages, raw (500 mg/kg), tomato juice (115 mg/L), vinegar (100 mg/L), wine (300 mg/L)

224   Potassium metabisulphite

Source   Manufactured from sulphur dioxide and potash.

Function   Potassium bisulphite has only 58% of the potency of sulphur dioxide. Dry, corrosive powder. Anti-fungal and anti-bacterial agent and antioxidant. Sulphites prevent both enzymic browning in fruit and vegetables and non-enzymic browning during processing of foods such as cooking meat or baking bread, biscuits and cakes. Sulphites prevent ascorbic acid (vitamin C) from being destroyed in fruit and fruit juice. However, sulphites destroy thiamine (vitamin B1).

Properties I have found that cooking with wine that contains sulphur dioxide removes all of the thiamine from the food. I would suggest that sulphur dioxide should not be allowed in sausages as this product is a source of thiamine.

Sulphites in foods have been implicated in initiating an asthma attack. Beverages such as wine have been blamed on asthma attacks. However, double blind clinical trials have recently been carried out by Professor Vally in Western Australia and asthmatics intolerant to wine seem to have diminished histamine degradation probably based on a deficiency of diamine oxidase. Acetaldehyde and amines such as histamine seem to be the cause of the attacks.

ADI 0–0.7 mg/kg body weight

Used in The ANZFS code suggests that a good manufacturing practice is to use no more than 350 mg/kg food.

In many cases manufacturers use far less than the recommended levels and sulphur dioxide and sulphites are destroyed rapidly by reducing sugars. For example, wine makers generally use only 50 parts per million of sulphur dioxide or sulphites in the initial stages of fermentation.

beer (25 mg/L), ginger beer (115 mg/L), canned fish (30 mg/kg), cider (200 mg/L), cheese (300 mg/kg), crystallised fruit (280 mg/kg), dried fruit (3 g/kg), dehydrated beans (750 mg/kg), dehydrated peas (200 mg/kg), dehydrated potatoes (500 mg/kg), flavoured cordials (230 mg/L), fruit drinks (115 mg/L), fruit juices (115 mg/L), fruit juice drinks (115 mg/L), gelatine (750 mg/kg), low-joule jams (285 mg/kg), pickles (750 mg/kg), soft drinks (115 mg/L), sausages, raw (500 mg/kg), tomato juice (115 mg/L), vinegar (100 mg/L), wine (300 mg/L)

225   Potassium sulphite

Source   Manufactured by adding potassium hydroxide to sulphurous acid.

Function   Potassium sulphite has only 45% of the potency of sulphur dioxide. Dry corrosive powder. Anti-fungal and anti-bacterial agent and antioxidant. Sulphites prevent both enzymic browning in fruit and vegetables and non-enzymic browning during processing of foods such as cooking meat or baking bread, biscuits and cakes. Sulphites prevent ascorbic acid (vitamin C) from being destroyed in fruit and fruit juice. However, sulphites destroy thiamine (vitamin B1).

Properties   I have found that cooking with wine that contains sulphur dioxide removes all of the thiamine from the food. I would suggest that sulphur dioxide should not be allowed in sausages as this product is a source of thiamine.

Sulphites have been implicated in initiating an asthma attack. Beverages such as wine have been blamed on asthma attacks. However, double blind clinical trials have recently been carried out by Professor Vally in Western Australia and asthmatics intolerant to wine seem to have diminished histamine degradation probably based on a deficiency of diamine oxidase. Acetaldehyde and amines such as histamine seem to be the cause of the attacks.

ADI   0–0.7 mg/kg body weight

Used in   The ANZFS code suggests that a good manufacturing practice is to use no more than 350 mg/kg food.

In many cases manufacturers use far less than the recommended levels and sulphur dioxide and sulphites are destroyed rapidly by reducing sugars. For example, wine makers generally use only 50 parts per million of sulphur dioxide or sulphites in the initial stages of fermentation.

beer (25 mg/L), ginger beer (115 mg/L), canned fish (30 mg/kg), cider (200 mg/L), cheese (300 mg/kg), crystallised fruit (280 mg/kg), dried fruit (3 g/kg), dehydrated beans (750 mg/kg), dehydrated peas (200 mg/kg), dehydrated potatoes (500 mg/kg), flavoured cordials (230 mg/L), fruit drinks (115 mg/L), fruit juices (115 mg/L), fruit juice drinks (115 mg/L), gelatine (750 mg/kg), low-joule jams (285 mg/kg), pickles (750 mg/kg), soft drinks (115 mg/L), sausages, raw (500 mg/kg), tomato juice (115 mg/L), vinegar (100 mg/L), wine (300 mg/L)

228   Potassium bisulphite

Source   Manufactured from potash and sulphur dioxide.

Function   Potassium bisulphite has only 63% of the potency of sulphur dioxide. Dry, corrosive powder. Anti-fungal and anti-bacterial agent and antioxidant. Sulphites prevent both enzymic browning in fruit and vegetables and non-enzymic browning during processing of foods such as cooking meat or baking bread, biscuits and cakes. Sulphites prevent ascorbic acid (vitamin C) from being destroyed in fruit and fruit juice. However, sulphites destroy thiamine (vitamin B1).

Properties   I have found that cooking with wine that contains sulphur dioxide removes all of the thiamine from the food. I would suggest that sulphur dioxide should not be allowed in sausages as this product is a source of thiamine.

Sulphites have been implicated in initiating an asthma attack. Beverages such as wine have been blamed on asthma attacks. However, double blind clinical trials have recently been carried out by Professor Vally in Western Australia and asthmatics intolerant to wine seem to have diminished histamine degradation probably based on a deficiency of diamine oxidase. Acetaldehyde and amines such as histamine seem to be the cause of the attacks.

ADI 0–0.7 mg/kg body weight

Used in The ANZFS code suggests that a good manufacturing practice is to use no more than 350 mg/kg food.

In many cases manufacturers use far less than the recommended levels and sulphur dioxide and sulphites are destroyed rapidly by reducing sugars. For example, wine makers generally use only 50 parts per million of sulphur dioxide or sulphites in the initial stages of fermentation.

beer (25 mg/L), ginger beer (115 mg/L), canned fish (30 mg/kg), cider (200 mg/L), cheese (300 mg/kg), crystallised fruit (280 mg/kg), dried fruit (3 g/kg), dehydrated beans (750 mg/kg), dehydrated peas (200 mg/kg), dehydrated potatoes (500 mg/kg), flavoured cordials (230 mg/L), fruit drinks (115 mg/L), fruit juices (115 mg/L), fruit juice drinks (115 mg/L), gelatine (750 mg/kg), low-joule jams (285 mg/kg), pickles (750 mg/kg), soft drinks (115 mg/L), sausages, raw (500 mg/kg), tomato juice (115 mg/L), vinegar (100 mg/L), wine (300 mg/L)

234 Nisin

Source Nisin is a low molecular weight antimicrobial peptide manufactured from selected strains of *Lactococcus lactis*, a common lactic acid-producing bacterium. It was discovered naturally occurring in many cheeses.

Function	Antimicrobial with an antibiotic like action (bacteriocin). Nisin is effective against a wide range of Gram-positive pathogenic bacteria (as vegetative cells as well as spores). Stable in processed acid foods.
Properties	No adverse effects
ADI	33,000 units/kg body weight, (0–0.25 mg/kg body weight)
Used in	cheese, cheese spreads, dips, pâté

235　Natamycin or Pimaricin

Source	Manufactured from fermentation using specific *Lactic* or *Subtilis bacteria.*
Function	Anti-bacterial agent with an antibiotic like action (bacteriocin). Natamycin is effective against pathogenic gram positive bacteria such as *Clostridium botulinum.* Stable during processing of foods.
Properties	There have been some concerns about bacteria becoming resistant or cross resistant to natamycin if it is over-used. According to the World Health Organisation, toxicological studies on natamycin or pimaricin were carried out and "Information available on the metabolism of pimaricin suggests it is not absorbed to a significant extent from the gastrointestinal tract. The only adverse effects found in animal studies were a decrease in food intake with a decrease in the rate of body-weight gain. The dog appeared to be more sensitive than the rat, the response appearing in dogs with doses of the order of 10 mg/kg/day. In man mild gastrointestinal symptoms begin to appear at daily dosage levels of about 5 mg/kg, although much higher dosage levels have been taken without ill-effects being observed. Adequate studies have demonstrated neither adverse effects on reproduction nor any carcinogenic,

mutagenic or teratogenic potential."

ADI 33,000 units/kg body weight (0–0.3 mg/kg body weight)

Used in cheese, savoury spreads, dips, sauces, mustard, horseradish cream

242 Dimethyl dicarbonate

Source Manufactured from two molecules of methanol and two molecules of carbon dioxide.

Function Broad antimicrobial range of action against yeasts, mould, fungi, and bacteria. It is unstable in aqueous solution but is an effective sterilising agent in only a few seconds and breaks down almost immediately after addition to beverages into methanol and carbon dioxide.

Properties The amounts of methanol formed by dimethyl dicarbonate in foods (120 parts per million) are of the same order as found in fruit juice and wine.

ADI 0–1.2 mg/kg body weight

Used in wine (250 mg/L), beer, fruit juices, fruit juice drinks

249 Potassium nitrite

Source Naturally occurring salt.

Function White powder, readily soluble in water. It is used as a preservative as well as a fixative for the red colour of ham, bacon and salami. The myoglobin pigments are converted to nitroso-met-myoglobin which is a bright red colour stable to processing and long term storage. Nitrites destroy pathogenic *E-coli* and *Clostridium botulinum* bacteria that are responsible for many deaths each year from consumption of meat products processed without nitrite.

Properties   Nitrites are formed by the action of bacteria in the mouth on salivary nitrate. They are thought to act synergistically with hydrochloric acid in the stomach in fighting food poisoning bacteria.

There has been concern over the use of nitrites in foods. Nitrite can combine with amines to form nitroso-amines which are among the most common cancer causing compounds (carcinogens). In many countries where relatively large amounts of nitrites are consumed, the incidence of oesophageal and stomach cancer is high. Infants less than six months of age cannot metabolise nitrites and they have been known to "fix" the haemoglobin in the blood, preventing the red blood cells from carrying oxygen, which has resulted in "chemical asphyxiation". However, nitrites destroy the more harmful pathogenic bacteria that can grow in meat products and food scientists have discovered that using vitamin C together with very low levels of nitrates and nitrites still preserves the food and nitroso-amines do not form.

ADI   0–0.2 mg/kg body weight

Used in   corned meats, cured, pickled or salted (125 mg/kg), canned cured meats (125 mg/kg), salami (125 mg/kg), mettwurst (125 mg/kg), bacon (125 mg/kg), ham (125 mg/kg)

250   Sodium nitrite

Source   Naturally occurring salt.

Function   White powder, readily soluble in water. It is used as a preservative as well as a fixative for the red colour of ham, bacon and salami. The myoglobin pigments are converted to nitroso-met-myoglobin which is a bright red colour stable to processing and long term storage. Nitrites destroy pathogenic *E-coli* and *Clostridium botulinum* bacteria that are responsible for many deaths each year from consumption of meat products processed without nitrite.

Properties Nitrites are formed by the action of bacteria in the mouth on salivary nitrate. They are thought to act synergistically with hydrochloric acid in the stomach in fighting food poisoning bacteria.

There has been concern over the use of nitrites in foods. Nitrite can combine with amines to form nitroso-amines which are among the most common cancer-causing compounds (carcinogens). In many countries where relatively large amounts of nitrites are consumed, the incidence of oesophageal and stomach cancer is high. Infants less than 6 months of age cannot metabolise nitrites and they have been known to "fix" the haemoglobin in the blood, preventing the red blood cells from carrying oxygen, which has resulted in "chemical asphyxiation". However, nitrites destroy the more harmful pathogenic bacteria that can grow in meat products and food scientists have discovered that using vitamin C together with very low levels of nitrates and nitrites still preserves the food and nitroso-amines do not form.

ADI 0–0.2 mg/kg body weight

Used in corned meats, cured, pickled or salted (125 mg/kg), canned cured meats (125 mg/kg), salami (125 mg/kg), mettwurst (125 mg/kg), bacon (125 mg/kg), ham (125 mg/kg)

251 Sodium nitrate

Source Naturally occurring salt.

Function White powder, readily soluble in water. Nitrate is converted to nitrites by bacteria in food. It is used as a preservative as well as a fixative for the red colour of ham, bacon and salami. The myoglobin pigments are converted to nitroso-met-myoglobin which is a bright red colour stable to processing and long term storage. Nitrites destroy pathogenic *E-coli* and *Clostridium botulinum* bacteria that are responsible for many deaths each year from consumption of meat products processed without nitrite.

Properties Nitrites are formed by the action of bacteria in the mouth on salivary nitrate. They are thought to act synergistically with hydrochloric acid in the stomach in fighting food poisoning bacteria.

There has been concern over the use of nitrites in foods. Nitrite can combine with amines to form nitroso-amines which are among the most common cancer-causing compounds (carcinogens). In many countries where relatively large amounts of nitrites are consumed, the incidence of oesophageal and stomach cancer is high. Infants less than 6 months of age cannot metabolise nitrites and they have been known to "fix" the haemoglobin in the blood, preventing the red blood cells from carrying oxygen, which has resulted in "chemical asphyxiation". However, nitrites destroy the more harmful pathogenic bacteria that can grow in meat products and food scientists have discovered that using vitamin C together with very low levels of nitrates and nitrites still preserves the food and nitroso-amines do not form.

ADI 0–0.2 mg/kg body weight

Used in corned meats, cured, pickled or salted (125 mg/kg), canned cured meats (125 mg/kg), salami (125 mg/kg), mettwurst (125 mg/kg), bacon (125 mg/kg), ham (125 mg/kg)

252 Potassium nitrate or saltpetre

Source Naturally occurring salt.

Function White powder, readily soluble in water. Nitrate is converted to nitrites by bacteria in food. It is used as a preservative as well as a fixative for the red colour of ham, bacon and salami. The myoglobin pigments are converted to nitroso-met-myoglobin which is a bright red colour stable to processing and long term storage. Nitrites destroy pathogenic *E-coli* and *Clostridium botulinum* bacteria that are responsible for many deaths each year from consumption of meat products processed without nitrite.

Properties Nitrites are formed by the action of bacteria in the mouth on salivary nitrate. They are thought to act synergistically with hydrochloric acid in the stomach in fighting food poisoning bacteria.

There has been concern over the use of nitrites in foods. Nitrite can combine with amines to form nitroso-amines which are among the most common cancer-causing compounds (carcinogens). In many countries where relatively large amounts of nitrites are consumed, the incidence of oesophageal and stomach cancer is high. Infants less than 6 months of age cannot metabolise nitrites and they have been known to "fix" the haemoglobin in the blood, preventing the red blood cells from carrying oxygen, which has resulted in "chemical asphyxiation". However, nitrites destroy the more harmful pathogenic bacteria that can grow in meat products and food scientists have discovered that using vitamin C together with very low levels of nitrates and nitrites still preserves the food and nitroso-amines do not form.

ADI 0–0.2 mg/kg body weight

Used in corned meats, cured, pickled or salted (125 mg/kg), canned cured meats (125 mg/kg), salami (125 mg/kg), mettwurst (125 mg/kg), bacon (125 mg/kg), ham (125 mg/kg)

260   Acetic acid, glacial

Source   Manufactured from methanol and carbon monoxide or oxidation of ethanol. Dilute solutions of acetic acid are formed naturally by aceto bacterial action on wine or beer in the presence of oxygen. The bacteria arrive naturally on the legs of "vinegar" flies that are attracted to wine or beer.

Function   Viscous liquid that imparts a pleasant sour acidic taste to many pickles and sauces. Acetic acid is antimicrobial because of its acidity and the undissociated molecule is effective against moulds and bacteria.

Properties In foods acetic acid is used at a concentration of only 2% and it is easily metabolised by the body to give energy and carbon dioxide. There have been many health claims that acetic acid can benefit digestion and "burn off" unwanted fat, but there is no scientific evidence to support these claims.

ADI   No ADI

Used in   pickles, relishes, dips, sauces, cheese, chutneys, marinades

261   Potassium acetate or Potassium diacetate

Source   Manufactured by adding potassium hydroxide to acetic acid.

Function   Maintains natural plant colours during processing and storage. It is also a buffering agent, being the salt of a weak acid, it has a high pH.

Properties No adverse affects

ADI   No ADI

Used in   pickles, relishes, dips, sauces, cheese, chutneys, marinades

262   Sodium acetate

Source   Manufactured by adding caustic soda to acetic acid.

Function   Mildly alkaline. Used as a buffer to maintain pH and retain colour of plant products.

Properties No adverse effects

ADI   No ADI

Used in   pickles, relishes, dips, sauces, cheese, chutneys, marinades

263   Calcium acetate

Source   Manufactured by the addition of lime to acetic acid.

Function   Relatively insoluble in foods but acts as a mould inhibitor and prevents "ropiness" in beer, bread and cider.

Properties No adverse affects

ADI   No ADI

Used in   pickles, relishes, dips, sauces, cheese, chutneys, marinades

264   Ammonium acetate

Source   Manufactured by treating acetic acid with liquid ammonia.

Function   Used as a buffer to control the pH of food.

Properties No adverse effects at levels used in foods.

ADI   No ADI

Used in   pickles, relishes, dips, sauces, cheese (flavoured), chutneys, marinades

270   Lactic acid

Source   Produced commercially from fermentation of a carbohydrate source such as sugar cane by bacteria such as *Lactobacillus bulgaricus* or *Bacillus acidilacti*. Lactic acid occurs naturally in sour milk or yoghurt. Bacteria are added to many wines to convert the harsh malic acid to the milder tasting lactic acid.

Function   Preserves food and acts as an acidulant. It imparts a pleasant taste to foods.

Properties   May cause diarrhoea in infants who cannot metabolise lactic acid, otherwise there are no adverse effects.

ADI   No ADI

Used in   yoghurt, salami, confectionery, sauces, sourdough bread

280   Propionic acid

Source   Manufactured from ethylene, water and carbon monoxide using catalysts. Propionic acid naturally occurs in alcoholic beverages and is formed during digestion of fat and bacteria in the rumen of cattle and sheep.

Fermentation technology is also used to manufacture propionic acid using *Propionibacterium acidipropionici* with corn syrup and molasses as the carbon sources to produce propionic acid together with acetic acid and succinic acid as by-products, via the dicarboxylic acid pathway.

Function   Liquid, very soluble in fat and water. Food preservative. Prevents "ropiness" in bread and beer. Food scientists have found that adding phosphoric acid to foods has a synergistic affect on the anti-fungal properties of propionic acid and less propionic acid needs to be added to foods.

Properties No adverse effects proven, but concern among Australian mothers who know of Sue Dengate's studies.

ADI 0–6 mg/kg body weight

Used in bread (1,000 mg/kg), Christmas puddings, baked goods, pitta bread

281 Sodium propionate

Source Manufactured by adding caustic soda to propionic acid. Naturally occurs in fermented foods such as wine, beer, olives and chocolate and bacteria in the rumen of cattle and sheep.

Function White powder, very soluble in water. Preservative with particular effectiveness against moulds and other fungi that grow on the surface of foods. Sodium propionate is also effective anti-fungal agent and bacteria that form "ropes" in bread and cider (*Bacillus mesentericus* and *Bacillus subtilus*).

Properties No adverse effects proven, but concern among Australian mothers who know of Sue Dengate's studies.

ADI 0–6 mg/kg body weight

Used in baked products, confectionery, frostings, poultry and pig feeds

282 Calcium propionate

Source Manufactured by adding lime to propionic acid. Occurs naturally during fermentation of beer, wine and bacteria in the rumen of cattle and sheep.

Function   White powder very soluble in water. Effective anti-fungal agent and bacteria that form "ropes" in bread and cider (*Bacillus mesentericus* and *Bacillus subtilus*).

Properties No adverse effects proven, but concern among Australian mothers who know of Sue Dengate's studies.

ADI   0–6 mg/kg body weight

Used in   pet and stock feeds, bread

283   Potassium propionate

Source   Manufactured by adding potassium hydroxide to propionic acid. Occurs naturally during fermentation of beer, wine and bacteria in the rumen of cattle and sheep.

Function   White powder very soluble in water. Effective anti-fungal agent and bacteria that form "ropes" in bread and cider (*Bacillus mesentericus* and *Bacillus subtilus*).

Properties No adverse effects proven, but concern among Australian mothers who know of Sue Dengate's studies.

ADI   0–6 mg/kg body weight

Used in   pastry, cakes, bread, rolls, confectionery, soft drinks

290   Carbon dioxide

Source   Produced from natural underground deposits. Some carbon dioxide is sold as a by-product of the brewing industry but it contains volatile impurities from the fermentation and must be purified.

Function   Propellant in pressurised cans. Preservative by excluding oxygen from food, preventing spoilage and pathogenic bacteria and moulds growing and lowering the pH of foods by producing carbonic acid. Carbon dioxide is also used to slow down the ripening process of fruit such as apples by modifying the atmosphere around the fruit either in warehouses or in packaging.

Properties No adverse effects in food but carbon dioxide is a dangerous gas in enclosed spaces, particularly in wineries and breweries where it is formed during fermentation. It is a colourless gas and can anaesthetise and asphyxiate workers. By law anyone working near carbon dioxide must be tethered by a belt and rope to someone else to prevent an accident.

ADI No ADI

Used in soft drinks, mineral water, alcoholic carbonated drinks, canned pressurised cream and non-stick oils, confectionery, packaged fresh salads and fruit

296   DL-Malic acid or Malic acid

Source White powder very soluble in water. Malic acid is found naturally as two identical formulae but as optically different forms (D and L enantiomers). It is found in apples, pears and berry fruit.

Function Acidulant and flavour additive (tart taste).

Properties No adverse effects with pure malic acid but there must be no maleic acid present as this acid is a nephro- (kidney) toxin.

ADI No ADI

Used in wines, fruit juice drinks, confectionery, soup mixes, sauces, burrito seasoning

297   Fumaric acid or allomaleic acid

Source Manufactured from maleic acid.

Function White powder that is sparingly soluble in water. Imparts a sour, acid taste to foods (five times sourer than citric acid). Used to inhibit malo-lactic bacteria in wines (0.1%). Fumaric acid destroys the disulphide bond in gluten, the protein that gives a loaf of bread volume. This makes the dough more elastic. It is also used in sourdough breads to make them sourer. Fumaric acid works synergistically with benzoic acid in preserving foods.

Properties No adverse effects

ADI No ADI

Used in fruit juice drinks, bread (rye and sourdough), wine, ginger beer

300 ANTIOXIDANTS, MORE FOOD ACIDS AND MINERAL SALTS

300 Ascorbic acid or vitamin C

Source White powder very soluble in water. Naturally occurring as the L-enantiomer as a white powder with an acidic, astringent taste. Found in fresh fruit and vegetables. Oranges contain about 35 mg of ascorbic acid per 100 gm, which is about the recommended daily allowance for good health. The Australian native fruit, Cape gooseberry has ten times the amount of ascorbic acid that is found in oranges. Destroyed by heat, enzymes (ascorbic acid oxidase), light and oxygen. Ascorbic acid is essential for all cells in the body. In particular it helps iron absorption from the small intestine and the synthesis of cartilage, bones, blood vessels, skin and teeth. A deficiency in ascorbic acid results in the disease "scurvy" which has symptoms of tiredness, loose teeth, bleeding gums, poor connective tissue, wounds that do not heal and eventually leads to death.

The most expensive forms of commercially available ascorbic acid are extracted from fresh fruit and are marketed as "natural", but there is no chemical difference in the cheapest form of ascorbic acid produced using electro-dialysis and fermentation of glucose by bacteria.

Function Antioxidant, bread improver, fortification of food additive, curing aid (helps maintain the colour stability of processed meats such as bacon, ham and salami). Prevents enzymic browning. Oxygen scavenger in packaged foods.

Properties No adverse effect as it is a vitamin. Some advocates suggest that ascorbic acid in large amounts (up to 10 gm/day!) "cure" the common cold but research studies have shown that it reduces the symptoms of a cold by acting as an antihistamine and these excessive amounts have given some people kidney stones or the tablets of ascorbic acid have blocked the small intestine.

ADI No ADI

Used in fresh fruit salad, fruit juices, fruit juice drinks, wine, fresh salads, cured meats, bread, frozen seafood, breakfast cereals

301   Sodium ascorbate

Source Manufactured by adding caustic soda to ascorbic acid.

Function Antioxidant, vitamin C, colour stabiliser in cured meats.

Properties No adverse effects

ADI No ADI

Used in fresh fruit salad, fruit juices, fruit juice drinks, wine, fresh salads, cured meats, bread, frozen seafood, breakfast cereals

302   Calcium ascorbate

Source   Manufactured by treating an ascorbic acid solution with lime.

Function   Used as an antioxidant and a source of vitamin C.

Properties No adverse effects at the concentrations used in food.

ADI   No ADI

Used in   fresh fruit salad, fruit juices, fruit juice drinks, wine, fresh salads, cured meats, bread, frozen seafood, breakfast cereals

303   Potassium ascorbate

Source   Manufactured by adding potassium hydroxide to ascorbic acid.

Function   Antioxidant, vitamin C, prevents enzymic browning in cut fruit and vegetables, stabilises colour in cured processed meat.

Properties No adverse effect

ADI   No ADI

Used in   fresh fruit salad, fruit juices, fruit juice drinks, wine, fresh salads, cured meats, bread, frozen seafood, breakfast cereals

304   Ascorbyl palmitate

Source   Manufactured by esterifying palmitic acid and ascorbic acid.

Function   Fat soluble liquid that is an antioxidant (binds oxygen), prevents non-enzymic oxidation in fruit and vegetables and stabilises the colour of cured processed meats such as salami, bacon and ham.

Acts synergistically with other antioxidants in preventing autoxidation of cooking oils at high processing temperatures.

Properties No adverse effects

ADI 0–1.25 mg/kg body weight

Used in cooking oils, margarine, nut meal, essential oils, salad oils, mayonnaise

306 Tocopherols concentrate, mixed

Source A mixture of α, γ and δ tocopherols. Produced by organic synthesis.

Function Colourless liquid soluble in fat but not water. They are incorporated into foods in pure fats or emulsions of water and fat, for example, margarine. Prevents oxidation of fat by quenching the chain reaction of free radicals with singlet oxygen. The tocopherols are vitamin E, which, together with selenium is essential in preventing oxidation of polyunsaturated fats, phospholipids and vitamin A in cell membranes in the body. Martha Clare Morris from the Rush Institute for Healthy Aging in Atlanta, Georgia, found in 2005 that the tocopherols from foods reduced the incidence of Alzheimer's disease in an aged population.

Properties No adverse effects

ADI 0.15–2 mg/kg body weight

Used in dips, spreads, margarine, mayonnaise, cooking oils, cooking fats, salad oils

307 α-Tocopherol

Source Produced by organic synthesis. Fat soluble liquid.

Function Antioxidant and vitamin E. The clinical results of the effects of vitamin E as a cancer preventive agent have been inconsistent. All published clinical trials with vitamin E have used α-tocopherol. Recent epidemiological, experimental and molecular studies suggest that α-tocopherol may be a more potent chemo-preventive form of vitamin E compared to the more-studied α-tocopherol.

Properties No adverse effects

ADI 0–1.25 mg/kg body weight

Used in dips, spreads, margarine, mayonnaise, cooking oils, cooking fats, salad oils

308 γ-Tocopherol

Source Produced by organic synthesis. Fat soluble liquid.

Function Antioxidant and vitamin E.

Properties No adverse effects.

ADI 0–1.25 mg/kg body weight

Used in dips, spreads, margarine, mayonnaise, cooking oils, cooking fats, salad oils

309 δ-Tocopherol

Source Produced by organic synthesis. Fat soluble liquid.

Function Antioxidant and vitamin E.

Properties No adverse effects

ADI 0–1.25 mg/kg body weight

Used in dips, spreads, margarine, mayonnaise, cooking oils, cooking fats, salad oils

310   Propyl gallate

Source   A white, crystalline, odourless, solid with a slightly bitter taste. It is manufactured by esterifying propyl alcohol with gallic acid, extracted from hazelnut shells. It can also be synthesised by biotechnology using *Aspergillus blanc*.

Function   Antioxidant. Works synergistically with citric acid. Propyl gallate quenches free radicals that oxidise fats. It is readily destroyed by heat. Propyl gallate is volatile and it is used in the packaging material of potato chips and breakfast cereals so that it can permeate the food and prevent oxidation.

Properties According to the World Health Organisation, "With one exception, in long-term studies in rats, gallates caused no demonstrable ill effects when fed at a level of 0.2%; in one investigation, however, this level resulted in hypochromic anaemia. It seems likely that this may have been due to interference with iron absorption, but the cause was not established. Haematological effects were carefully examined in a number of other investigations and no abnormalities were seen."

ADI   0–2.5 mg/kg body weight

Used in   dips, spreads, margarine (100 ppm), mayonnaise, cooking oils (1,000 ppm), cooking fats, salad oils

311   Octyl gallate

Source   A white, crystalline, odourless, solid. Manufactured by esterifying octyl alcohol with gallic acid derived from hazelnut shells.

Function   Antioxidant octyl gallate is volatile and it is used in the packaging material of potato chips and breakfast cereals so that it can permeate the food and prevent oxidation.

Properties No adverse effects

ADI No ADI

Used in dips, spreads, margarine, mayonnaise, cooking oils, cooking fats, salad oils

312 Dodecyl gallate

Source Manufactured by esterifying dodecyl alcohol with gallic acid derived from hazelnut shells.

Function Antioxidant. Dodecyl gallate is volatile and it is used in the packaging material of potato chips and breakfast cereals so that it can permeate the food and prevent oxidation.

Properties No adverse effects

ADI No ADI

Used in dairy blends of butter and oils, dips, spreads, margarine (9,100 ppm), mayonnaise, cooking oils (1,000 ppm), cooking fats, salad oils

315 Erythorbic acid

Source Manufactured by organic synthesis.

Function Antioxidant, oxygen scavenger and aids in the development and stability during storage of the colour of processed meat products such as bacon, salami and ham. Erythorbic acid is the iso-isomer of ascorbic acid but it has only one twentieth of the activity of vitamin C as ascorbic acid. However, it works synergistically with nitrates and nitrites, reducing the amount needed for colour development and stability thus reducing the possibility of carcinogenic nitroso-amines forming in foods.

Properties No adverse effects

ADI   No ADI

Used in   fresh fruit salad, fruit juices, fruit juice drinks, wine, fresh salads, cured meats, bread, frozen seafood, breakfast cereals

316   Sodium erythorbate

Source   Manufactured by organic synthesis.

Function   Antioxidant, oxygen scavenger and aids in the development and stability during storage of the colour of processed meat products such as bacon, salami and ham. Erythorbic acid is the iso-isomer of ascorbic acid but it has only one twentieth of the activity of vitamin C as ascorbic acid. However, it works synergistically with nitrates and nitrites, reducing the amount needed for colour development and stability thus reducing the possibility of carcinogenic nitroso-amines forming in foods.

Properties   No adverse effects

ADI   No ADI

Used in   fresh fruit salad, fruit juices, fruit juice drinks, wine, fresh salads, cured meats, bread, frozen seafood, breakfast cereals

319   tert-Butylhydroquinone

Source   Cream coloured solid. Manufactured from by-products of petroleum.

Function   Antioxidant. Not allowed in infant foods. Quenches free radicals so that they do not oxidise fats in foods. It is volatile and it is used in the packaging material of potato chips and breakfast cereals so that it can permeate the food and prevent oxidation.

Properties   No adverse effects

| ADI | 0–0.2 mg/kg body weight |
| Used in | dips, spreads, margarine, mayonnaise, cooking oils, cooking fats, salad oils |

320   Butylated hydroxyanisole

Source	White fat soluble solid. Manufactured from by-products of petroleum.
Function	Antioxidant. Not allowed in infant foods. Quenches free radicals so that they do not oxidise fats in foods. It is volatile and it is used in the packaging material of potato chips and breakfast cereals so that it can permeate the food and prevent oxidation.
Properties	No adverse reactions at the concentrations used in food.
ADI	0–0.5 mg/kg body weight
Used in	dips, spreads, margarine, mayonnaise, cooking oils, cooking fats, salad oils

321   Butylated hydroxytoluene

Source	Manufactured from by-products of petroleum.
Function	Not allowed in infant foods. Antioxidant. Quenches free radicals so that they do not oxidise fats in foods. It is volatile and it is used in the packaging material of potato chips and breakfast cereals so that it can permeate the food and prevent oxidation.
Properties	No adverse effects
ADI	No ADI
Used in	dips, spreads, margarine, mayonnaise, cooking oils, cooking fats, salad oils

322   Lecithin

Source   Phospho-lipid fractions of legumes and present in all membranes of the human body. Extracted as a by-product of soy bean oil processing. Naturally occurring in egg yolks.

Function   In the human body it forms structures in the cell membranes, protecting the cells. Lecithin is responsible for the functional properties of eggs in cake-making and emulsion formation of mayonnaise. In the food industry it is primarily used as an emulsifier, allowing the hydrophobic surface of fats to combine with water. It also allows different phases of ingredients to form stable emulsions such as air, fat, water (ice cream): water, meat solids, fat and water (sausages).

Properties   No adverse effects

ADI   No ADI

Used in   baked products, mayonnaise, low-fat salad dressings, margarine, chocolate, confectionery, dips

325   Sodium lactate

Source   Manufactured by adding caustic soda to lactic acid produced by continuous production of lactic acid by immobilised *Bifidobacterium longum* (*B. longum*) using cheese whey as a substrate.

Function   Acidity regulator, humectant, bulking agent.

Properties   No adverse effects

ADI   No ADI

Used in   yoghurt, salami, confectionery, sauces, sourdough bread

326   Potassium lactate

Source   Manufactured by adding potassium hydroxide to lactic acid produced by continuous production of lactic acid by immobilised *Bifidobacterium longum (B. longum)* using cheese whey as a substrate.

Function   Acidity regulator, humectant, bulking agent.

Properties   No adverse effects

ADI   No ADI

Used in   pet foods, yoghurt, salami, confectionery, sauces, sourdough bread

327   Calcium lactate

Source   Manufactured by adding lime to lactic acid produced by continuous production of lactic acid by immobilised *Bifidobacterium longum (B. longum)* using cheese whey as a substrate.

Function   Acidity regulator and humectant in semi-dried foods such as pet foods.

Properties   No adverse effects

ADI   No ADI

Used in   pet foods, yoghurt, salami, confectionery, sauces, sourdough bread

328   Ammonium lactate

Source   Manufactured by adding ammonia to lactic acid produced by continuous production of lactic acid by immobilised *Bifidobacterium longum (B. longum)* using cheese whey as a substrate.

Function   Acidity regulator

Properties   No adverse effects

ADI   No ADI

Used in   yoghurt, salami, confectionery, sauces, sourdough bread

329   Magnesium lactate

Source   Manufactured by adding magnesium hydroxide to lactic acid produced by continuous production of lactic acid by immobilised *Bifidobacterium longum* (*B. longum*) using cheese whey as a substrate.

Function   Acidity regulator.

Properties   No adverse reactions at the concentrations used in food.

ADI   No ADI

Used in   yoghurt, salami, confectionery, sauces, crumpets

330   Citric acid

Source   Manufactured by biotechnology using sucrose from molasses and *Aspergillus niger* fungi.

Function   Acidic taste enhancer. Acidity regulator and acts synergistically with antioxidants to reduce fat oxidation. Citric acid removes copper and ferrous molecules that catalyse autoxidation of fats.

Properties   No adverse effects, but taken in excess citric acid can upset the stomach.

ADI   No ADI

Used in   fruit juice drinks, soft drinks, wine, dips, pâté, sauces, curry pastes, jelly, processed cheese

331   Sodium citrate

Source   Manufactured by adding caustic soda to citric acid.

Function   Acts as a buffering agent controlling pH and binds ferrous and cuprous ions that catalyse the autoxidation of fats.

Properties   No adverse effects

ADI   No ADI

Used in   fruit juice drinks, jams, ice confections, wine, dips, pâté, sauces, curry pastes, jelly, processed cheese

332   Potassium citrate

Source   Manufactured by adding potassium hydroxide to citric acid.

Function   Acts as a buffering agent controlling pH and binds ferrous and cuprous ions that catalyse the autoxidation of fats. Emulsion stabiliser.

Properties   No adverse effects

ADI   No ADI

Used in   fruit juice drinks, jams, ice confections, dips, pâté, sauces, curry pastes, jelly, processed cheese, sausages

333   Calcium citrate (mono, di and tri)

Source   Manufactured by adding different amounts of lime to citric acid.

Function   Acts as a buffering agent controlling pH and binds ferrous and cuprous ions that catalyse the autoxidation of fats. Acts as an emulsifying agent in sausage manufacturing.

Properties   No adverse effects

ADI   No ADI

Used in   fruit juice drinks, jams, ice confections, wine, dips, pâté, sauces, curry pastes, jelly, sausages, processed cheese

334   Tartaric acid (L+)

Source   Tartaric acid is found naturally in many acid fruits. There is also a D, L form of tartaric acid made from biotechnology using fungi fermentation but it cannot be used in beverages as it can precipitate out and form a cloudy haze of calcium tartrate.

It is extracted from fruit pulp and as a by-product of the wine industry. Potassium tartrate is removed from white wine to stabilise it and acid is added to convert the potassium tartrate to tartaric acid.

Function   Acidity regulator in soft drinks, wine, jellies and baked products. Tartaric acid is also an antioxidant because it sequesters cuprous and ferrous ions that catalyse autoxidation of fats.

Properties No adverse effects

ADI   0–30 mg/kg body weight

Used in   confectionery, wine, soft drinks, baked products, jelly, fruit juice drinks, cordials

335   Sodium tartrate (L+)

Source   Manufactured by adding caustic soda to tartaric acid.

Function   Acidity regulator emulsifier in fat and water emulsions. Sodium tartrate sequesters cuprous and ferrous.

Properties No adverse effects

ADI   0–30 mg/kg body weight

Used in   confectionery, wine, soft drinks, baked products, jelly, fruit juice drinks, cordials

336   Potassium tartrate or Potassium acid tartrate

Source   Known to the Greeks and Romans as tartar. Louis Pasteur studied potassium tartrate crystals which he found to be asymmetric. He found that the crystals could rotate light to the left. It is a by-product of the wine industry. Pure crystals of potassium tartrate precipitate out or adhere to the walls of storage vessels during "chill proofing" of white wine.

Function   Used as an acidity regulator, acts as a buffer (pH stabiliser) in beverages.

Properties No adverse effects

ADI   0–30 mg/kg body weight

Used in   confectionery, wine, soft drinks, baked products, jelly, fruit juice drinks, cordials

337   Potassium sodium tartrate

Source   Manufactured by adding equal molar amounts of caustic soda and potassium hydroxide to tartaric acid.

Function   Used as an acidity regulator, acts as a buffer (pH stabiliser) foods.

Properties No adverse effects

ADI   0–30 mg/kg body weight

Used in   powdered cake mixes, powdered spices, dried yeast

338   Phosphoric acid

Source Phosphoric acid exists either as a crystal or clear liquid. It is a colourless, odourless liquid, or a thick, unstable crystalline solid.

Function Acidifier. Provides a pleasant acid taste to foods and beverages such as cola soft drinks.

Properties Nutritionists have been concerned about by the high levels of phosphoric acid and phosphates in the foods of children. If there is too much phosphorus and not enough calcium in the diet then the body draws on the calcium from the bones. Too much phosphorus from cola drinks can cause the bones to become brittle and prone to fracture or in later life to lead to osteoporosis ("porous bones"). The plasma levels of calcium and phosphorus must be balanced for a number of important biochemical functions in the body.

ADI No ADI

Maximum allowable levels
70 mg (as phosphorus)/kg body weight

Used in cola soft drinks (600 mg/L), cottage cheese, cream cheese, pressure pack cream, processed meat products

339   Sodium phosphate

Source Manufactured by adding caustic soda to phosphoric acid.

Function Acidity regulator, emulsifier, stabiliser.

Properties No adverse effects. See phosphoric acid (338).

ADI No ADI

Maximum allowable levels
70 mg (as phosphorus)/kg body weight

Used in   cottage cheese, cream cheese, pressure pack cream, processed meat products

340   Potassium phosphate

Source   Manufactured by adding potassium hydroxide to phosphoric acid.

Function   Acidity regulator, emulsifier, stabiliser.

Properties   No adverse effects. See phosphoric acid (338).

ADI   No ADI

Maximum allowable levels
70 mg (as phosphorus)/kg body weight

Used in   cottage cheese, cream cheese, pressure pack cream, processed meat products

341   Calcium phosphate

Source   Manufactured by adding lime to phosphoric acid.

Function   Acidity regulator, emulsifier, stabiliser, anti-caking agent.

Properties   No adverse effects. See phosphoric acid (338).

ADI   No ADI

Maximum allowable levels
70 mg (as phosphorus)/kg body weight

Used in   cottage cheese, cream cheese, pressure pack cream, processed meat products

342   Ammonium phosphate

Source   Manufactured by injecting ammonia into a solution of phosphoric acid.

Function   Acidity regulator.

Properties   No adverse effects. See phosphoric acid (338).

ADI   No ADI

Maximum allowable levels
70 mg (as phosphorus)/kg body weight

Used in   cottage cheese, cream cheese, pressure pack cream, processed meat products

343   Magnesium phosphate

Source   Manufactured by adding magnesium oxide to phosphoric acid.

Function   Acidity regulator, anti-caking agent, yeast food.

Properties   No adverse effects. See phosphoric acid (338).

ADI   No ADI

Maximum allowable levels
70 mg (as phosphorus)/kg body weight

Used in   cottage cheese, cream cheese, pressure pack cream, processed meat products, yeast

349   Ammonium malate

Source   Manufactured by injecting ammonia into a solution of malic acid.

Function   Acidity regulator

Properties   No adverse effects

ADI   No ADI

Used in   fruit juice drinks, cordials, fruit and cheese dips, sauces

350   Sodium malate

Source   Manufactured by adding caustic soda to malic acid.

Function   Acidity regulator, humectant.

Properties   No adverse effects

ADI   No ADI

Used in   fruit juice drinks, cordials, fruit and cheese dips, sauces, wine

351   Potassium malate

Source   Manufactured by adding potassium hydroxide to malic acid.

Function   Acidity regulator

Properties   No adverse effects

ADI   No ADI

Used in   fruit juice drinks, cordials, fruit and cheese dips, sauces

352   Calcium malate

Source   Manufactured by adding lime to malic acid.

Function   Acidity regulator.

Properties   No adverse effects

ADI   No ADI

Used in   fruit juice drinks, cordials, fruit and cheese dips, sauces

353   Metatartaric acid

Source   Manufactured from tartaric acid.

Function   Acidity regulator and fining agent to remove excess calcium in wine.

Properties No adverse effects

ADI   No ADI

Used in   wine (< 100mg/L)

354   Calcium tartrate

Source   Manufactured by adding lime to tartaric acid.

Function   Acidity regulator.

Properties No adverse effects

ADI   No ADI

Used in   baked goods, pâté

355   Adipic acid

Source   Appears naturally in plant cells. Manufactured by nitric acid oxidation of cyclohexanol.

Function   Acidity regulator and buffer.

Properties No adverse effects

ADI   0–5 mg/kg body weight

Used in   reduced sodium foods, salt (sodium chloride) replacers

357   Potassium adipate

Source   Manufactured by adding potassium hydroxide to adipic acid.

Function   Acidity regulator, buffer and salt replacer.

Properties No adverse effects

ADI   No ADI

Used in   reduced sodium foods, salt (sodium chloride)
                replacers

359   Ammonium adipate

Source   Manufactured by injecting ammonia gas into a
                solution of adipic acid.

Function   Acidity regulator, buffer and salt replacer.

Properties No adverse effects, but people with liver or kidney
                diseases should avoid it.

ADI   0–5 mg/kg body weight

Used in   reduced sodium foods, salt (sodium chloride)
                replacers

363   Succinic acid

Source   Occurs in all living cells and fermented foods such as
                cheese and wine. Manufactured from acetic acid.

Function   Acidity regulator.

Properties No adverse reactions at the concentrations used in
                foods.

ADI   0–5 mg/kg body weight

Used in   cake mixes, wine, liqueurs, baked goods

365   Sodium fumarate

Source   Manufactured by adding caustic soda to fumaric acid.

Function   Acidity regulator, spice and seasoning additive.
                Destroys malo-lactic bacteria in wine. Acts
                synergistically with sodium benzoate. Firming agent
                with pectin and gelatine gels.

Properties No adverse effects

ADI 0–5 mg/kg body weight

Used in wine, cheese spreads, dips, jelly, jams, marmalades, fruit juice drinks

366 Potassium fumarate

Source Manufactured by adding potassium hydroxide to fumaric acid.

Function Acidity regulator, spice and seasoning additive. Destroys malo-lactic bacteria in wine. Acts synergistically with sodium benzoate. Firming agent with pectin and gelatine gels.

Properties No adverse effects

ADI 0–5 mg/kg body weight

Used in wine, cheese spreads, dips, jelly, jams, marmalades, fruit juice drinks

367 Calcium fumarate

Source Manufactured by adding caustic soda to fumaric acid.

Function Acidity regulator, spice and seasoning additive. Destroys malo-lactic bacteria in wine. Acts synergistically with sodium benzoate. Firming agent with pectin and gelatine gels.

Properties No adverse effects

ADI 0–5 mg/kg body weight

Used in wine, cheese spreads, dips, jelly, jams, marmalades, fruit juice drinks

368   Ammonium fumarate

Source   Manufactured by injecting ammonia into solutions of fumaric acid.

Function   Acidity regulator, spice and seasoning additive. Destroys malo-lactic bacteria in wine. Acts synergistically with sodium benzoate. Firming agent with pectin and gelatine gels.

Properties   No adverse effects

ADI   0–5 mg/kg body weight

Used in   wine, cheese spreads, dips, jelly, jams, marmalades, fruit juice drinks

380   Ammonium citrate or triammonium citrate

Source   Manufactured by injecting ammonia gas into a citric acid solution.

Function   Acidulation, buffer and sequestrant agent. Acts synergistically with antioxidants to prevent autoxidation of fats.

Properties   No adverse effects

ADI   No ADI

Used in   cheese spreads, processed cheese

381   Ferric ammonium citrate

Source   Manufactured by adding ferric chloride and ammonia to citric acid. Brown, green powder.

Function   Acidity regulator, anti-caking agent and used to fortify foods with iron.

Properties   No adverse effects

ADI   0–1 mg/kg body weight

Used in   breakfast cereals, dry package cake mixes, salt, spice mixes

385   Calcium disodium ethylenediaminetetraacetate or calcium disodium EDTA

Source   Manufactured from ethylene, ammonia and acetic anhydride.

Function   EDTA removes metallic ions by strongly binding (sequesters) them and starving micro-organisms of essential nutrients so that they die. Because EDTA sequesters cuprous and ferrous ions it prevents ion catalysed free radical oxidation of fats. It therefore acts synergistically with antioxidants. EDTA binds other mineral ions that discolour food.

Properties No adverse effects for concentrations used in foods. It is used to treat lead poisoning.

ADI   0–2.5 mg/kg body weight

Used in   mayonnaise, canned vegetables, margarine, salad dressings, baked goods, confectionery, beer, stout, cooking oils, cheese spreads, dips, processed meats

400 THICKENING AGENTS, VEGETABLE GUMS, EMULSIFIERS AND THEIR MINERAL SALTS

Most of the gums are derived from plants so that they can be consumed by people who are vegans, vegetarians or have religious restrictions. Gums are usually added in combination with other gums or starches to increase the functional properties. A starch/gum ingredient system offers several advantages. A mixture stabilises an emulsion at high temperatures of processing and during freeze storage. Starch maintains an emulsion at temperatures below 20°C but breaks down at higher temperatures, while most gums are stable at high temperatures. Selecting the right gum usually on the advice of the supplier maintains the emulsion.

Starch and gum combinations also help to minimize syneresis. This is useful in freeze-thaw applications where starches tend to release moisture upon thawing. By adding a gum to the system, excess moisture released by the starch is subsequently absorbed by the gum and product integrity is maintained. A frozen, baked item, for example, could be ruined if its custard filling released too much moisture when thawed. A blend of a starch and a gum in the filling would eliminate this problem.

400   Alginic acid

Source   Naturally occurring in seaweed. Extracted with hot alkaline water from specific types of brown seaweed (*Phaeophyceae*). It is a hydrophilic colloidal polysaccharide copolymer consisting mainly of residues of 1, 4-linked D-mannuronic acid and 1, 4-linked L-glucuronic acid.

Function   Thickening agent used with other hydrocolloid gels to form stable gel products.

Properties   No adverse effects at levels used in foods. High intakes can bind essential minerals in the intestine leading to mineral deficiencies and high concentrations cause flatulence and bloating due to fermentation by the gastrointestinal bacteria. It is a laxative.

ADI   0–25 mg/kg body weight

Used in puddings, ice cream, yoghurt, frozen desserts, thickened cream, glazes for buns, cakes and pastry, low-fat salad dressings, mayonnaise

401   Sodium alginate

Source   Manufactured by adding caustic soda to alginic acid.

Function   Thickening agent used with other hydrocolloid gels to form stable gel products.

Properties No adverse effects at levels used in foods.
High intakes can bind essential minerals in the intestine leading to mineral deficiencies and high concentrations cause flatulence and bloating due to fermentation by the gastrointestinal bacteria. It is a laxative.

ADI   0–25 mg/kg body weight

Used in puddings, ice cream, yoghurt, frozen desserts, thickened cream, glazes for buns, cakes and pastry, low-fat salad dressings, mayonnaise

402   Potassium alginate

Source   Manufactured by adding potassium hydroxide to alginic acid.

Function   Thickening agent used with other hydrocolloid gels to form stable gel products.

Properties No adverse effects at levels used in foods.
High intakes can bind essential minerals in the

intestine leading to mineral deficiencies and high concentrations cause flatulence and bloating due to fermentation by the gastrointestinal bacteria. It is a laxative.

ADI   0–25 mg/kg body weight

Used in   puddings, ice cream, yoghurt, frozen desserts, thickened cream, glazes for buns, cakes and pastry, low-fat salad dressings, mayonnaise

403   Ammonium alginate

Source   Manufactured by injecting ammonia gas into solutions of alginic acid.

Function   Thickening agent used with other hydrocolloid gels to form stable gel products.

Properties No adverse effects at levels used in foods. High intakes can bind essential minerals in the intestine leading to mineral deficiencies.

ADI   0–25 mg/kg body weight

Used in   puddings, ice cream, yoghurt, frozen desserts, thickened cream, glazes for buns, cakes and pastry, low-fat salad dressings, mayonnaise

404   Calcium alginate

Source   Manufactured by adding lime to alginic acid.

Function   Thickening agent used with other hydrocolloid gels to form stable gel products.

Properties No adverse effects at levels used in foods. High intakes can bind essential minerals in the intestine leading to mineral deficiencies.

ADI   0–25 mg/kg body weight

Used in puddings, ice cream, yoghurt, frozen desserts, thickened cream, glazes for buns, cakes and pastry, low-fat salad dressings, mayonnaise

405   Propylene glycol alginate

Source Manufactured by esterifying alginic acid with propyl alcohol and glycol.

Function Thickening agent used with other hydrocolloid gels to form stable gel products.

Properties No adverse effects at levels used in foods. High intakes can bind essential minerals in the intestine leading to mineral deficiencies. Professor Anderson of Edinburgh University studied the effects of propylene glycol on humans and found that the ingestion of propylene glycol alginate at a high level for 23 days caused no adverse dietary or physiological effects; in particular, the enzymatic and other sensitive indicators of adverse toxicological effects remained unchanged, but high concentrations cause flatulence and bloating due to fermentation by the gastrointestinal bacteria. It is a laxative.

ADI 0–25 mg/kg body weight

Used in frozen ices, beer (maintains foam), puddings, ice cream, yoghurt, frozen desserts, thickened cream, glazes for buns, cakes and pastry, low-fat salad dressings, mayonnaise

406   Agar

Source Sourced from seaweed in New Zealand and India.

Function Thickening agent used with other hydrocolloid gels to form stable gel products.

Properties Not digested. It passes through the body unchanged.

Promotes the proliferation of probiotics ("good bacteria"). No adverse effects at levels used in foods. High intakes can bind essential minerals in the intestine leading to mineral deficiencies and high concentrations cause flatulence and bloating due to fermentation by the gastrointestinal bacteria. It is a laxative.

ADI   0–25 mg/kg body weight

Used in   puddings, ice cream, yoghurt, frozen desserts, thickened cream, glazes for buns, cakes and pastry, low-fat salad dressings, mayonnaise

407   Carrageenan or Irish moss

Source   Naturally occurring and is obtained by extracting red seaweed (*Chondrus crispus*) with hot alkaline water.

Function Gelling and thickening agent, imparts a good texture in desserts and frozen milk products. Acts as an emulsifier in processed meat products.

Properties No adverse effects. There was some confusion about carrageenan which was thought to be toxic as it was called "poligeenan". Poligeenan is a toxin formed by chemically breaking down carageenan and this is used for industrial purposes.

ADI   No ADI

Used in   frozen desserts, low-fat yoghurt and ice cream, processed meats, confectionery, cough lollies

407a   Processed eucheuma seaweed or iota carageenan

Source   Naturally occurring and is obtained by extracting red seaweed (*Eucheuma spinosum* species) with hot alkaline water.

Function   Gelling and thickening agent, imparts a good texture in desserts and frozen milk products. Acts as an emulsifier in processed meat products.

Properties   No adverse effects. According to the World Health Organisation who studied eucheuma seaweed at "concentrations of 0, 0.5, 1.5, or 5% in the diet, as well as conventionally processed carrageenan from these two sources at 5% in the diet. At the highest concentrations in the diet, the intakes of the seaweeds were equal to 4300 and 5000 mg/kg body weight per day, respectively, for male and female rats fed the material from *E. cottonii* and to 4500 and 5100 mg/kg body weight per day, respectively, for male and female rats fed the material from *E. spinosum*. No adverse effects were noted in the study. The changes observed during the course of feeding the highest concentration of processed Eucheuma seaweed from these two sources, most notably an increase in the relative weights of the full and empty caecum, were considered to be the consequence of accumulation of poorly absorbed material in the caecum and to be of no toxicological significance. There was no indication that the effects of the processed Eucheuma seaweeds differ from those of conventionally prepared carrageenans from the same seaweed species.

Processed Eucheuma seaweed derived from either *E. cottonii* or *E. spinosum* was not mutagenic in well-conducted assays for reverse mutation in *Salmonella typhimurium* strains. The Committee considered that no further studies of genotoxicity were required." High concentrations cause flatulence and bloating due to fermentation by the gastrointestinal bacteria. It is a laxative.

ADI   No ADI

Used in   frozen desserts, low-fat yoghurt and ice cream, processed meats, confectionery, cough lollies

409   Arabinogalactan or Larch gum

Source   Derived by extracting the wood of the Western larch tree (*Larix occidentalis* species).

Function   Thickener, gelling agent. Stabiliser of emulsions such as low-fat salad dressing. Used in conjunction with other gums.

Properties   No adverse effects. Arabinogalactan has positive effects as a medicine for diseases such as otitis media and it has been shown to work synergistically with anti cancer drugs that prevent metastasis (the spreading of cancer from one organ to the other), but high concentrations cause flatulence and bloating due to fermentation by the gastrointestinal bacteria. It is a laxative.

ADI   No ADI

Used in   frozen desserts, low-fat yoghurt, ice cream, processed meats, confectionery

410   Locust bean gum or Carob bean gum

Source   Originally used on the bandages that were used to preserve mummies in Egypt, this gum is extracted from the seeds of the leguminous European carob tree *Ceratonia siliqua*. In the Bible it is referred to as St John's bread.

Function   Gelling agent and thickener. It forms stable emulsion gels with oil and water which makes it ideal for salad dressings. It gives a good mouth feel to liquids.

Properties   No adverse effects but studies have shown that dietary locust bean gum can reduce plasma cholesterol and has a beneficial effect on gut flora, but high concentrations cause flatulence and bloating due to fermentation by the gastrointestinal bacteria. It is a laxative.

ADI   No ADI

Used in   salad dressings, low-fat salad dressings, mayonnaise, dips, spreads, frozen desserts, low-fat yoghurt, ice cream, processed meats, confectionery

412   Guar gum

Source   Guar gum is extracted guar bean seed (*Cyamopsis tetragonolobus*) ground endosperm. The guar plant is leguminous and mainly grown in India and Pakistan.

Function   Guar gum is a polysaccharide made up of galactan and mannan units which have the properties of forming hydrophilic gels that thicken foods, giving them a pleasant mouth feel. They also stabilise emulsions so that mayonnaise does not separate into oil and water phases.

Properties   No adverse effects in food but in the pure form it was once used as a dietary weight reduction aid, filling the stomach preventing hunger. However, the Food and Drug Agency in the US banned its use as there were some consumers who had blocked intestines! High concentrations cause flatulence and bloating, due to fermentation by the gastrointestinal bacteria. It is a laxative.

ADI   No ADI

Used in   salad dressings, low-kilojoule salad dressings, mayonnaise, dips, spreads, frozen desserts, low-fat yoghurt, ice cream, processed meats, confectionery

413   Tragacanth gum

Source   Extracted from the sap of *Astragalus gummifer*, *A. adscendens* and *A. microcephalus*. The sap is a gummy, mucilaginous product. "Tragacanth" comes from the appearance of the exuded gum, which forms strips similar in appearance to a goat horn ("tragos", Greek for goat and "akantha" for horn).

Function   Thickener and emulsion stabiliser in foods with oil and water.

Properties   No adverse effects but like other plant gums it reduces plasma cholesterol and has a favourable effect on probiotics in the gastrointestinal tract, but high concentrations cause flatulence and bloating due to fermentation by the gastrointestinal bacteria. It is a laxative.

ADI   No ADI

Used in   salad dressings, low-kilojoule salad dressings, mayonnaise, dips, spreads, frozen desserts, low-fat yoghurt, ice cream, processed meats, confectionery

414   Acacia or gum Arabic

Source   Water-soluble gum obtained by extracting species of the acacia tree, especially *Acacia senegal* and *A. arabica* , in the gum belt of Africa such as Northern Mauritania, West Niger, Nigeria, Senegal, Chad, Zimbabwe, Kenya, Mali and Sudan.

Function   Emulsion stabiliser and thickener, giving a good mouth feel to beverages. Used in conjunction with other gums. Used as a sugar and nutrient coating cereal bars and snack foods. For bakery products, the gum's binding and emulsification properties aid in the formulation of icings and frostings as well as baked goods like cakes and buns.

Properties   No adverse effects but like other plant gums, it reduces plasma cholesterol and has a favourable effect on probiotics in the gastrointestinal tract, but high concentrations cause flatulence and bloating due to fermentation by the gastrointestinal bacteria. It is a laxative.

ADI   No ADI

Used in   salad dressings, low-kilojoule salad dressings, mayonnaise, dips, spreads, frozen desserts, low-fat yoghurt, ice cream, processed meats, confectionery

415   Xanthan gum

Source   This gum was discovered when scientists found certain bacteria produced it, which allowed them to stick onto plants, making them hard to remove. This "sticky" polymer is manufactured by aerobic fermentation using the bacteria *Xanthomonas campestris*. Xanthan gum is a D-glucopyranose glucan with chains of linked D-mannopyranose, D-glucuronic acid and D-mannopyranose on every second unit.

Function   Stabiliser, inhibiting emulsion breakdown which would lead to a poor appearance of margarines and spreads (oil and water phases separate). It sticks to food so that it is used in edible packaging and toppings and icings on baked products. Enhanced mouth feel is obtained from an increase in viscosity as the gum absorbs water. It also allows pulp in fruit juice and fruit juice drinks to remain suspended and increases baking volume in flour products.

Properties   No known adverse effects. Xanthan gum passes almost unchanged through the body and allows probiotic bacteria to proliferate in the gastrointestinal tract, but high concentrations cause flatulence and bloating due to fermentation by the gastrointestinal bacteria. It is a laxative.

ADI   No ADI

Used in   baked goods, icings, fruit juices, fruit juice drinks, salad dressings, low-kilojoule salad dressings, mayonnaise, dips, spreads, frozen desserts, low-fat yoghurt, ice cream, processed meats, confectionery

416   Karaya gum

Source   Dried exudation of the Indian tree *Sterculia urens*.

Function   Used as a thickening and gelling agent in foods with other gums.

Properties   No adverse effects, but high concentrations cause flatulence and bloating due to fermentation by the gastrointestinal bacteria. It is a laxative.

ADI   No ADI

Used in   puddings, ice cream, yoghurt, frozen desserts, thickened cream, glazes for buns, cakes and pastry, low-fat salad dressings, mayonnaise

418   Gellan gum

Source   This polymer is manufactured by aerobic fermentation using the bacteria *Sphingomonas elodea*.

Function   Thickener, stabiliser and gelling agent, particularly suited to suspending fine solids in soy and chocolate drinks.

Properties   No adverse effects, but high concentrations cause flatulence and bloating due to fermentation by the gastrointestinal bacteria. It is a laxative.

ADI   No ADI

Used in   soy drinks, chocolate milkshakes, fruit juice drinks, coconut milk

420 SWEETENERS, HUMECTANTS, EMULSIFIERS

420   Sorbitol or sorbitol syrup

Source   Sorbitol, a polyol (sugar alcohol), naturally occurs in the tree berries and many fruit. It is manufactured by hydrogenation of glucose and is available in both liquid and crystalline form.

Function   Sweetener, humectant, emulsifier. Sorbitol is about 56% as sweet as table sugar but contains less than 60% of the kilojoules of sugar, making it a useful additive in diabetic foods. It has a pleasant, sweet and cool taste which is ideal for peppermint and spearmint lollies and toothpaste. It does not form brown pigments during processing as sugars do (non-enzymic browning) so that it is useful as a sugar replacer in baked goods. It absorbs water, preventing foods from drying out so that it is used in some pre-cooked pie crusts

Properties   No adverse effects. Unlike sucrose, it does not encourage teeth-decaying bacteria.

ADI   No ADI

Used in   confectionery (peppermint and spearmint lollies), low-energy foods, carbohydrate modified foods, pastry crusts, baked goods

421   Mannitol or manna sugar

Source   Naturally occurs in foods such as celery. Manufactured by the fermentation of sugars glucose and maltose by bacteria *Lactobacillus intermedius*.

Function   Sweetener, humectant. It has only 50% of the kilojoules of sugar and because it does not raise insulin levels, it is ideal in diabetic foods and low-energy foods. Prevents confectionery from absorbing water and becoming sticky. It is used as a coating for lollies.

Properties No adverse effects. Unlike sucrose, it does not encourage teeth decaying. It can have a laxative effect.

ADI No ADI

Used in confectionery as a coating material, low-energy foods

422 Glycerin or glycerine or glycerol

Source Manufactured by hydrolysing vegetable and animal fats to fatty acids and glycerol. The salts of the fatty acids become soap and the glycerol is separated from it.

Function Humectant allowing foods to contain higher levels of water without spoiling. This is because the water is bound to the glycerol and is unavailable to bacteria and moulds and it cannot undergo many chemical reactions. Glycerin has the same energy content as sugars (16.5 kJ/g) but it does not raise insulin levels in the blood so that it is used in some diabetic foods. It gives a pleasant mouth feel to drinks such as liqueurs.

Properties No adverse effects

ADI No ADI

Used in semi-moist foods such as pet foods and fruit cakes, diabetic foods, crystallised fruit, dried fruit, liqueurs, alcoholic spirits

430 FATTY ACID POLYOL EMULSIFIERS

These are a group of excellent emulsifiers which are used in a wide range of foods. Food scientists calculate the emulsification power by the HLB System (hydrophilic-lipophilic balance system).

The theoretical values of HLB range from 1 to approximately 50. A surface-active agent can be given value to measure its relative hydrophilic and lipophilic property.

For polyhydric alcohol and fatty acid esters:

$$HLB = 20 (1 - S/Ac)$$

where S is the saponification number and
Ac is the acid number of the acid.

When S is undetermined:

$$HLB = (O + W) / 5$$

where O is the weight percent of oxyethylene and
W is the weight percent of polyhydric alcohol.

When oxyethylene is the only hydrophilic group:

$$HLB = O / 5$$

Generic or Chemical name	HLB
Sorbitan trioleate	1.8
Propylene glycol mono-stearate	3.4
Glycerol mono-stearate	3.8
Propylene glycol mono-laurate	4.5
Sorbitan mono-stearate	4.7
Glyceryl mono-stearate (self-emulsifying)	5.5
Sorbitan mono-laurate	8.6
Polyoxyehtylene-4-lauryl ether	9.5
Polyethylene glycol 400 mono-stearate	11.6
Polyoxyethylene-4-sorbitan mono-laurate	13.3
Polyoxyethylene-20-sorbitan mono-palmitate	15.6
Polyoxyethylene-40-stearate	16.9
Sodium oleate	18.0
Sodium lauryl sulphate	40.0

The more hydrophilic emulsifiers have HLB values greater than 10, while the more lipophylic emulsifiers have HLB values from 1 to 10. As a general rule, emulsifiers with HLB values in the range of 4 to 7 will promote water in oil emulsions; values between 8 to 17 promote oil in water emulsions.

431 Polyethylene (40) stearate

Source   Mixture of mono- and distearate esters of macrogols (polyoxyethylene polymers) with an average length of the polymer chain equal to 40. Synthesised by esterifying polyethyl alcohols and stearic acid derived from beef fat.

Function   Emulsifier and anti-foaming agent (0.1%).

Properties   No adverse effects

ADI   0–25 mg/kg body weight

Used in   pharmaceuticals, confectionery, mayonnaise, low-energy salad dressings, malt extract, distilled spirits (anti-foam), sausage casings

433 Polysorbate 80 or Polyoxyethylene (20) sorbitan mono-oleate or Tween 80

Source   A mixture of sorbitol anhydride polymerised with ethylene oxide and oleic esters of sorbitol with an average length of the polymer chain equal to 80.

Function   Emulsifier and anti-foaming agent.

Properties   No adverse effects

ADI   No ADI

Used in   bread, chocolate, shortenings

435 Polysorbate 60 or Polyoxyethylene (20) sorbitan monostearate or Tween 60

Source   A mixture of sorbitol anhydride polymerised with ethylene oxide and oleic esters of sorbitol with an average length of the polymer chain equal to 60.

Function   Emulsifier and anti-foaming agent (0.1%).

Properties   No adverse effects

ADI   0–25 mg/kg body weight

Used in   pharmaceuticals, confectionery, mayonnaise, low-energy salad dressings, malt extract, distilled spirits (anti-foam), sausage casings

436 Polysorbate 65 Polyoxyethylene (20) or sorbitan tristearate or Tween 65

Source   A mixture of sorbitol anhydride polymerised with ethylene oxide and oleic esters of sorbitol with an average length of the polymer chain equal to 65.

Function   Anti-foaming agent (0.1%) and emulsifier.

Properties   No adverse effects

ADI   0–25 mg/kg body weight

Used in   pharmaceuticals, confectionery, mayonnaise, low-energy salad dressings, malt extract, distilled spirits (anti-foam), sausage casings, cake mixes

440 Pectin

Source   Extracted from the cell walls of dicotyledonous plants. In combination with cellulose, it gives structure and rigidity to plant tissues. It is particularly abundant in apples, oranges and lemons. There are low and high methoxy-pectins which have different gel strengths and mouth feel.

Function	Thickener, stabiliser, gelling agent. High methoxy-pectins are very stable to thermal processing such as jam manufacturing and glazes on buns.
Properties	No adverse effects. Pectins bind heavy metals such as lead and mercury, aiding in their excretion from the gastro-intestinal tract. Pectins lower the glycemic index of foods, and lower plasma cholesterol.
ADI	No ADI
Used in	1 High methoxy-pectins: sugar jelly, jams, preserves, marmalades, milk drinks, glazes on baked products
	2 Low methoxyl-pectins: diabetic jelly, jams, preserves, marmalades

442   Ammonium salts of phosphatidic acid

Source	Manufactured by injecting ammonia into a solution of phosphatidic acid.
Function	Emulsifier, foaming agent, whipping agent.
Properties	According to the World Health Organisation, "The biochemical studies show that the ammonium salts of phosphatidic acids break down into normal food constituents. The available rat studies show this material to be non-toxic at the level of 6% in the diet, the highest concentration tested. A long-term study together with reproduction studies on one species were also carried out which showed no adverse effects."
ADI	0–30 mg/kg body weight
Used in	ice cream, puddings, yoghurt, cream, bread rolls, cacao products

444   Sucrose acetate isobutyrate

Source   Manufactured by esterifying sucrose with acetic and isobutyric acid.

Function   Emulsifier and stabiliser for flavouring compounds that are oil based and need to be incorporated into aqueous foods. Produces a haze in soft drinks such as bitter lemon.

Properties No adverse effects

ADI   0–20 mg/kg body weight

Used in   non-alcoholic drinks, essential oils, sauces, taco mixes, mustard

445   Glycerol esters of wood rosins

Source   Manufactured by extracting rosin from wood pulp and esterifying the acid groups with glycerol.

Function   Emulsifier, stabiliser. Used to make a haze in soft drinks. Allows essential oils to form an emulsion in foods.

Properties No adverse effects

ADI   0–25 mg/kg body weight

Used in   soft drinks, chewing gum, essential oils

450   Potassium pyrophosphate or Sodium acid pyrophosphate or Sodium pyrophosphate

Source   Manufactured by converting phosphoric acid to sodium ortho-phosphate and then heating this mixture at high temperatures.

Function   Emulsifiers, acidity regulators, colour stabilisers in processed meats. Dissolves myoglobin proteins in meat allowing them to form stable gels in salami and mettwurst sausages. Retains essential minerals such as iron in processed meat products.

Properties No adverse effects but high levels of phosphates in the diet may weaken bones (see phosphoric acid (338)).

ADI 0–30 mg/kg body weight

Maximum allowable levels
70 mg/ kg body weight (from all phosphorus sources)

Used in baking powder

451 Potassium tripolyphosphate or Sodium tripolyphosphate

Source Manufactured by fusing tripolyphosphoric acid (made from phosphoric acid) with caustic soda or potassium hydroxide.

Function Acidity regulator, buffer

Properties No adverse effects but high levels of phosphates in the diet may weaken bones (see phosphoric acid (338)).

ADI 0–30 mg/kg body weight

Maximum allowable levels
70 mg/ kg body weight (from all phosphorus sources)

Used in confectionery, mayonnaise, low-energy salad dressings, malt extract, distilled spirits (anti-foam), sausage casings

452 Potassium polymetaphosphate or Sodium metaphosphate, insoluble or Sodium polyphosphates, glassy

Source Natural deposits of polymetaphosphate (Graham's salt) are mined in China. The various salts are purified by recrystallisation from aqueous saturated solutions.

Function Buffer and yeast nutrient.

Properties No adverse effects but high levels of phosphates in the diet may weaken bones (see phosphoric acid (338)).

ADI 0–30 mg/kg body weight

Maximum allowable levels
70 mg/ kg body weight (from all phosphorus sources)

Used in cottage cheese, cream cheese, pressure pack cream, processed meat products, yeast

460   Cellulose microcrystalline and powdered

Source Manufactured as a by-product of the wood pulp industry by breaking down cellulose fibres with enzymes derived from fungi.

Function Anti-caking agent, bulking agent in low-energy foods and dietary fibre. Good thaw-refreeze properties.

Properties No adverse effects. As a dietary fibre it acts as a laxative and removes toxins from the gastrointestinal tract.

ADI No ADI

Used in cake mixes, gravy powders, low-energy foods, extruded foods, deep-fried foods, frozen prepared meals

461   Methyl cellulose

Source Manufactured as a by-product of the wood pulp industry by methylating cellulose fibres that have been extracted and broken down with enzymes derived from fungi.

Function   Thickener, stabiliser, emulsifier and fat extender. Good thaw-refreeze properties.

Properties No adverse effects. As a dietary fibre it acts as a laxative and removes toxins from the gastrointestinal tract.

ADI   No ADI

Used in   cake mixes, gravy powder, low-energy foods, low-fat products, extruded foods, deep-fried foods, frozen prepared meals

463   Hydroxypropyl cellulose

Source   Manufactured as a by-product of the wood pulp industry by hydroxy-propylating cellulose fibres with hydroxy-propyl groups.

Function   Thickener, stabiliser, emulsifier and fat extender. Good thaw-refreeze properties.

Properties No adverse effects. As a dietary fibre it acts as a laxative and removes toxins from the gastrointestinal tract.

ADI   No ADI

Used in   cake mixes, gravy powders, low-energy foods, low-fat foods, extruded foods, deep-fried foods, frozen prepared meals

464   Hydroxypropyl methylcellulose

Source   Manufactured as a by-product of the wood pulp industry by methylating and hydroxy propylating cellulose fibres with methyl and hydroxy propyl groups.

Function   Thickener, stabiliser, emulsifier and fat extender. Good thaw-refreeze properties.

Properties   No adverse effects. As a dietary fibre it acts as a laxative and removes toxins from the gastrointestinal tract.

ADI   No ADI

Used in   cake mixes, gravy powder, low-energy foods, low-fat foods, extruded foods, deep-fried foods, frozen prepared meals

465   Methyl ethyl cellulose

Source   Manufactured as a by-product of the wood pulp industry by breaking down cellulose fibres with enzymes derived from fungi and methylating and ethylating the hydroxy groups of cellulose.

Function   Thickener, stabiliser, emulsifier and foaming agent. Good thaw-refreeze properties.

Properties   No adverse effects. As a dietary fibre it acts as a laxative and removes toxins from the gastrointestinal tract.

ADI   No ADI

Used in   cake mixes, gravy powders, low-energy foods, extruded foods, deep-fried foods, frozen prepared meals

466   Sodium carboxymethylcellulose

Source   Manufactured as a by-product of the wood pulp industry by breaking down cellulose fibres with enzymes derived from fungi, methylating the cellulose and forming the sodium salt.

Function   Thickener, stabiliser and bulking agent in low-energy foods. Good thaw-refreeze properties.

Properties   No adverse effects. As a dietary fibre it acts

as a laxative and removes toxins from the
gastrointestinal tract.

ADI   No ADI

Used in   cake mixes, gravy powders, low-energy foods, soy
milk, low-energy foods, extruded foods, deep-fried
foods, frozen prepared meals

470   Aluminium, calcium, sodium, magnesium, potassium and ammonium salts of fatty acids

Source   Myristic, palmitic and stearic acids are naturally
occurring fatty acid components of animal tallow
and vegetable oils. The aluminium, calcium, sodium,
magnesium and ammonium salts can be made from
these fatty acids by the addition of the appropriate
oxides.

Function   Emulsifier, stabiliser and anti-caking agent.

Properties No adverse effects

ADI   No ADI

Used in   bread, cakes, pies, gravy mixes, dry cake mixes

471   Mono- and di-glycerides of fatty acids

Source   Manufactured by partial esterification of glycerol
with selected fatty acids.

Function   Emulsifier and stabiliser. Used to homogeneously
mix water and oil based foods by acting as a "bridge"
between hydrophobic (oil) and hydrophilic (aqueous)
groups. This also includes foam stability.

Properties No adverse effects

ADI   No ADI

Used in   artificial milk, confectionery, dairy products,
flavoured milks, baked goods, ice cream, frozen

desserts, margarine, mayonnaise, soup mixes, thickened cream

472a   Acetic and fatty acid esters of glycerol

Source   Manufactured by partial esterification of glycerol with acetic acid and selected fatty acids.

Function   Emulsifier and stabiliser. Used to homogeneously mix water and oil based foods by acting as a "bridge" between hydrophobic (oil) and hydrophilic (aqueous) groups. This also includes foam stability.

Properties   No adverse effects

ADI   No ADI

Used in   artificial milk, confectionery, dairy products, flavoured milk, baked goods, ice cream, frozen desserts, margarine, mayonnaise, soup mixes, thickened cream

472b   Lactic and fatty acid esters of glycerol

Source   Manufactured by partial esterification of glycerol with lactic acid and selected fatty acids.

Function   Emulsifier and stabiliser. Used to homogeneously mix water and oil based foods by acting as a "bridge" between hydrophobic (oil) and hydrophilic (aqueous) groups. This also includes foam stability.

Properties   No adverse effects

ADI   No ADI

Used in   artificial milk, confectionery, dairy products, flavoured milk, baked goods, ice cream, frozen desserts, margarine, mayonnaise, soup mixes, thickened cream

472c Citric and fatty acid esters of glycerol

Source Manufactured by partial esterification of glycerol with lactic acid and selected fatty acids.

Function Emulsifier and stabiliser. Used to homogeneously mix water and oil based foods by acting as a "bridge" between hydrophobic (oil) and hydrophilic (aqueous) groups. This also includes foam stability.

Properties No adverse effects

ADI No ADI

Used in artificial milk, confectionery, dairy products, flavoured milk, baked goods, ice cream, frozen desserts, margarine, mayonnaise, soup mixes, thickened cream

472e Diacetyltartaric and fatty acid esters of glycerol

Source Manufactured by partial esterification of glycerol with diacetyltartaric acid and selected fatty acids.

Function Emulsifier and stabiliser. Used to homogeneously mix water and oil based foods by acting as a "bridge" between hydrophobic (oil) and hydrophilic (aqueous) groups. This also includes foam stability.

Properties No adverse effects

ADI No ADI

Used in artificial milk, confectionery, dairy products, flavoured milk, baked goods, ice cream, frozen desserts, margarine, mayonnaise, soup mixes, thickened cream

472f Mixed tartaric, acetic and fatty acid esters of glycerol

Source Manufactured by partial esterification of glycerol with acetic, tartaric and selected fatty acids.

Function   Emulsifier and stabiliser. Used to homogeneously mix water and oil based foods by acting as a "bridge" between hydrophobic (oil) and hydrophilic (aqueous) groups. This also includes foam stability.

Properties No adverse effects

ADI   No ADI

Used in   artificial milk, confectionery, dairy products, flavoured milk, baked goods, ice cream, frozen desserts, margarine, mayonnaise, soup mixes, thickened cream

473   Sucrose esters of fatty acids

Source   Manufactured by partial esterification of sucrose with selected fatty acids.

Function   Emulsifier and stabiliser. Used to homogeneously mix water and oil based foods by acting as a "bridge" between hydrophobic (oil) and hydrophilic (aqueous) groups. This also includes foam stability.

Properties No adverse effects

ADI   0–10 mg/kg body weight.

Used in   artificial milk, confectionery, dairy products, flavoured milk, baked goods, ice cream, frozen desserts, margarine, mayonnaise, soup mixes, thickened cream

475   Polyglycerol esters of fatty acids

Source   Manufactured by partial esterification of polyglycerol with selected fatty acids.

Function   Emulsifier and stabiliser. Used to homogeneously mix water and oil based foods by acting as a "bridge"

between hydrophobic (oil) and hydrophilic (aqueous) groups. This also includes foam stability.

Properties No adverse effects

ADI 0–10 mg/kg body weight.

Used in artificial milk, confectionery, dairy products, flavoured milk, baked goods, ice cream, frozen desserts, margarine, mayonnaise, soup mixes, thickened cream

476 Polyglycerol esters of interesterified ricinoleic acid

Source Manufactured by esterification of polyglycerol with ricinoleic acid.

Function Emulsifier and stabiliser. Used to homogeneously mix water and oil based foods by acting as a "bridge" between hydrophobic (oil) and hydrophilic (aqueous) groups. This also includes foam stability.

Properties No adverse effects

ADI 0–10 mg/kg body weight.

Used in artificial milk, confectionery, dairy products, flavoured milk, baked goods, ice cream, frozen desserts, margarine, mayonnaise, soup mixes, thickened cream

477 Propylene glycol mono- and di-esters or Propylene glycol esters of fatty acids

Source Manufactured by partial esterification of propylene glycol with selected fatty acids.

Function Emulsifier and stabiliser. Used to homogeneously mix water and oil based foods by acting as a "bridge" between hydrophobic (oil) and hydrophilic (aqueous) groups. This also includes foam stability.

Properties No adverse effects

ADI 0–10 mg/kg body weight.

Used in artificial milk, confectionery, dairy products, flavoured milk, baked goods, ice cream, frozen desserts, margarine, mayonnaise, soup mixes, thickened cream

480 Dioctyl sodium sulphosuccinate

Source Manufactured by esterification of octyl alcohol with sulpho-succinic acid.

Function Emulsifier and stabiliser. Used to homogeneously mix water and oil based foods by acting as a "bridge" between hydrophobic (oil) and hydrophilic (aqueous) groups. This also includes foam stability.

Properties No adverse effects

ADI 0–10 mg/kg body weight.

Used in artificial milk, confectionery, dairy products, flavoured milk, baked goods, ice cream, frozen desserts, margarine, mayonnaise, soup mixes, thickened cream

481 Sodium lactylate or sodium oleyl lactylate or sodium stearoyl lactylate

Source Manufactured by esterification of lactyl alcohol with stearic acid from beef tallow and then forming the sodium salt with caustic soda.

Function Emulsifier and stabiliser. Used to homogeneously mix water and oil based foods by acting as a "bridge" between hydrophobic (oil) and hydrophilic (aqueous) groups. This also includes foam stability.

Properties No adverse effects

ADI 0–10 mg/kg body weight.

Used in   artificial milk, confectionery, dairy products, flavoured milk, baked goods, ice cream, frozen desserts, margarine, mayonnaise, soup mixes, thickened cream

482   Calcium lactylate or Calcium oleyl lactylate or Calcium stearoyl lactylate

Source   Manufactured by partial esterification of lactyl alcohol stearic and oleic fatty acids and then adding lime to obtain the calcium salt.

Function   Emulsifier and stabiliser. Used to homogeneously mix water and oil based foods by acting as a "bridge" between hydrophobic (oil) and hydrophilic (aqueous) groups. This also includes foam stability.

Properties No adverse effects

ADI   0–10 mg/kg body weight.

Used in   artificial milk, confectionery, dairy products, flavoured milk, baked goods, ice cream, frozen desserts, margarine, mayonnaise, soup mixes, thickened cream

491   Sorbitan monostearate

Source   Manufactured by esterification of equal molar amounts of sorbitol and stearic acid.

Function   Emulsifier and stabiliser. Used to homogeneously mix water and oil based foods by acting as a "bridge" between hydrophobic (oil) and hydrophilic (aqueous) groups. This also includes foam stability.

Properties No adverse effects

ADI   0–10 mg/kg body weight.

Used in   artificial milk, confectionery, dairy products, flavoured milk, baked goods, ice cream, frozen desserts, margarine, mayonnaise, soup mixes, thickened cream

492   Sorbitan tristearate

Source   Manufactured by esterification of one molar amount of sorbitol with three molar amounts of stearic acid.

Function   Emulsifier and stabiliser. Used to homogeneously mix water and oil based foods by acting as a "bridge" between hydrophobic (oil) and hydrophilic (aqueous) groups. This also includes foam stability. Sorbitan tristearate improves loaf volume in bread-making.

Properties   No adverse effects

ADI   0–10 mg/kg body weight.

Used in   artificial milk, confectionery, dairy products, flavoured milk, baked goods, ice cream, frozen desserts, margarine, mayonnaise, soup mixes, thickened cream

500 MINERAL SALTS AND ANTI-CAKING AGENTS

500   Sodium carbonate or Sodium bicarbonate

Source   Manufactured electrolytically from sea water or by the "Solvay" process where carbon dioxide is passed into a saturated solution of sodium chloride and ammonia. Ammonium carbonate is formed and this passes into ammonium hydrogen carbonate, which reacts with sodium chloride to form sodium hydrogen carbonate and ammonium chloride. Sodium hydrogen carbonate precipitates as a solid and is filtered off.

Function   Acidity regulator, raising agent, anti-caking agent.

Properties   No adverse effects

ADI   No ADI

Used in   cake mixes, confectionery, malt extract, self-raising flour, mayonnaise, soup mixes

501 Potassium carbonate

Source   Manufactured electrolytically from potassium chloride solution or by the "Solvay" process where carbon dioxide is passed into a saturated solution of potassium chloride and ammonia. Ammonium carbonate is formed and this passes into ammonium hydrogen carbonate, which reacts with potassium chloride to form sodium hydrogen carbonate and ammonium chloride. Sodium hydrogen carbonate precipitates as a solid and is filtered off.

Function   Acidity regulator, raising agent, anti-caking agent.

Properties   No adverse effects

ADI   No ADI

Used in   cake mixes, confectionery, malt extract, self-raising flour, mayonnaise, soup mixes

503 Ammonium bicarbonate or Ammonium hydrogen carbonate

Source   Manufactured by injecting ammonia into carbon dioxide solution.

Function   Acidity regulator, anti-caking agent.

Properties   No adverse effects

ADI   No ADI

Used in   cake mixes, confectionery, malt extract, self-raising flour, mayonnaise, soup mixes

504 Magnesium carbonate or magnesite

Source   Manufactured electrolytically with magnesium metal and carbon dioxide in a water solution. Occurs also as pure deposits as magnesite.

Function   Acidity regulator, anti-caking agent.

Properties   No adverse effects

ADI   No ADI

Used in   cake mixes, confectionery, malt extract, self-raising flour, mayonnaise, soup mixes

507   Hydrochloric acid

Source   Manufactured electrolytically from sea water. Naturally occurring as acid in the stomach that aids digestion of food.

Function   Acidity regulator.

Properties   No adverse effects at the levels used in foods.

ADI   No ADI

Used in   cottage cheese, tofu, cream cheese

508   Potassium chloride

Source   Occurs naturally as pure mineral deposits.

Function   Gelling agent and salt replacer.

Properties   No adverse effects

ADI   No ADI

Used in   low-sodium foods, salt replacers, jelly, jams, confectionery, glazes on baked goods.

509   Calcium chloride

Source   Manufactured as a by-product of the "Solvay" process and occurs as natural deposits.

Function   Firming agent and precipitate of protein gels. Used to fortify foods with calcium. Used in the brewing industry to accelerate yeast settling.

Properties No adverse effects

ADI No ADI

Used in tofu, malt extract, cottage cheese, canned tomatoes, chutney, fruit juices, bread, breakfast cereals

510   Ammonium chloride

Source Prepared by injecting ammonia into hydrochloric acid solution.

Function Bulking agent, yeast food together with phosphoric acid. Prevents hydrogen sulphide ("rotten egg" gas) forming in wine and beer.

Properties No adverse effects, but consumers with kidney or liver disease should avoid it.

ADI No ADI

Used in salt substitutes, beer, wine, flour for bread-making

511   Magnesium chloride

Source Manufactured by adding sulphuric acid to magnesium ammonium chloride hexahydrate.

Function Firming agent, colour stabiliser and nutrient.

Properties No adverse effects. Magnesium is an essential nutrient found in every cell of the body.

ADI No ADI

Used in beer, salt replacers, tofu, cottage cheese, cheese spreads

512 Stannous chloride

Source   Manufactured from tin ore and sulphuric acid.

Function   Antioxidant, flavouring agent and colour stabiliser.

Properties   No adverse effects. Although it has been suggested that ingested inorganic tin may undergo biomethylation to the more toxic forms of alkyl tin, there is no conclusive evidence that this occurs in experimental animals or man.

ADI   0–2 mg/kg body weight

Used in   canned beans, canned asparagus, tomato juice

514 Sodium sulphate

Source   Naturally occurs as mirabilite (Canada) and thenardite (Russia).

Function   Acidity regulator and as a food for brewing yeast.

Properties   No adverse effects

ADI   No ADI

Used in   brewing, colour pigment extender

515 Potassium sulphate

Source   Naturally occurs in a mixture of potassium, magnesium and calcium sulphate and is separated on a solubility and re-crystallisation basis.

Function   Acidity regulator and salt replacer.

Properties   No adverse effects

ADI   No ADI

Used in   confectionery, low-energy salad dressings, malt extract, salt replacements, low-sodium foods

516   Calcium sulphate

Source   Natural deposits are mined in Europe and America.

Function   Firming agent and used to fortify foods with calcium.

Properties   No adverse effects

ADI   No ADI

Used in   bread, milk, tofu, soy milk, cottage cheese, jelly, canned tomatoes, baking powder

518   Magnesium sulphate or Epsom salts or epsomite

Source   Natural deposits occur where sea waters have dried up in deposits of limestone.

Function   Firming agent and used to supply magnesium to yeast in the brewing industry and in infant food.

Properties   No adverse effects but it is a laxative.

ADI   No ADI

Used in   beer, bread, milk, tofu, soy milk, cottage cheese, jelly, canned tomatoes, baking powder, infant formulas

519   Cupric sulphate

Source   Manufactured by mixing copper ores with sulphuric acid. Occurs naturally as deposits of bright blue hydrocyanite and chalcanthite.

Function   Mineral salt and removes hydrogen sulphide ("rotten egg" gas) from wine.

Properties   No adverse effects but only 0.5 parts per million are used in wine.

ADI   No ADI

Used in   infant foods, wine

526   Calcium hydroxide

Source   Manufactured by adding water to lime (calcium oxide or "quick lime").

Function Acidity regulator, neutralises acid in fruit juice and wines from cold regions that develop too much acid. Used as a firming agent in fruit gels and in brewery mash water to give calcium ions that allow yeast to settle.

Properties No adverse effects

ADI   No ADI

Used in   bread, fruit jelly, beer, infant foods, wine

529   Calcium oxide or "quick lime"

Source   Manufactured by heating limestone to 500°C to drive off the carbon dioxide from calcium carbonate.

Function Acidity regulator.

Properties No adverse effects

ADI   No ADI

Used in   beer, canned peas, canned asparagus, fruit juices

530   Magnesium oxide

Source   Naturally occurring in an impure form. Purified by recrystallisation in water and drying well so that it absorbs water.

Function Anti-caking agent.

Properties No adverse effects, but in high doses it acts as a laxative.

ADI   No ADI

Used in   table salt, dry gravy mixes, canned peas, tofu

535 Sodium ferrocyanide or sodium hexacyanoferrate II

Source Manufactured from cyanic acid, caustic soda and ferrous sulphate.

Function Anti-caking agent.

Properties No adverse effects. The strong bonding within the molecules of sodium ferrocyanide prevents the release of the toxic cyanide.

ADI 0–0.025 mg/kg body weight

Used in salt (50 mg/kg)

536 Potassium ferrocyanide or potassium hexacyanoferrate II

Source Manufacture from caustic potash, ferrous sulphate and cyanic acid.

Function Anti-caking agent and used to remove iron and copper from canned corn where these metals cause off colours and in wine where these metals can cause an unsightly haze.

Properties No adverse effects. The strong bonding within the molecules of sodium ferrocyanide prevents the release of the toxic cyanide.

ADI 0–0.025 mg/kg body weight

Used in salt (50 mg/kg), wine, canned corn

541   Sodium aluminium phosphate

Source   Manufactured from phosphoric acid, aluminium and caustic soda.

Function   Acidity regulator, leavening agent and emulsifier.

Properties No adverse effects

ADI   0–0.6 mg/kg body weight

Used in   tacos, tortillas, specialty savoury biscuits

542   Bone phosphate or edible calcium phosphate of bone

Source   Manufactured from degreased abattoir bones that are heated to remove collagen protein.

Function   Used as anti-caking agent, emulsifier and nutrient.

Properties No adverse effects

ADI   No ADI

Used in   bread, dried milk, processed meat products

551   Silicon dioxide, amorphous

Source   Manufactured by grinding quartz or sand to a fine particle (< 100 micro metres) and boiling in hydrochloric acid to form a colloidal gel.

Function   Used as an anti-caking agent and suspending agent. The hard nature makes confectionery firm.

Properties No adverse effects because silicon dioxide passes straight through the body unchanged.

ADI   No ADI

Used in   confectionery, beer (aids clarification), wine (aids clarification), artificial milk, salt, salt substitutes

552   Calcium silicate

Source   Naturally occurring in the pure form as wollastonite
             in limestone deposits from which it is extracted.

Function   Used as an anti-caking agent and antacid.

Properties No adverse effects.

ADI   No ADI

Used in   salt, salt substitutes, antacid tablets

553   Magnesium silicate or Talc or French chalk

Source   Natural deposits occur throughout Australia.

Function   Used as an anti-caking agent, releasing agent.
             Filtering aid and dusting powder on confectionery.

Properties No adverse effects

ADI   No ADI

Used in   confectionery, chocolate, baking (releasing agent),
             chewing gum

554   Sodium aluminosilicate or analcite or natrolite

Source   Occurs naturally as pure deposits and can be
             manufactured from silica sand and gibbsite mineral.

Function   Used as an anti-caking agent.

Properties No adverse effects. At one time it was thought
             that aluminium salts were a neurotoxin because
             Alzheimer's disease sufferers had deposits of
             aluminium in their brains, but it is now known that
             only organic derivatives of aluminium are dangerous.

ADI   No ADI

Used in   artificial milk, table salt

555 Potassium aluminium silicate

Source   Occurs naturally as pure deposits of amazonite and as a type of feldspar mineral Microcline. It can also be manufactured from silica sand, caustic potash and aluminium by fusion at high temperatures.

Function   Used as an anti-caking agent.

Properties   No adverse effects. At one time it was thought that aluminium salts were a neurotoxin because Alzheimer's disease sufferers had deposits of aluminium in their brains, but it is now known that only organic derivatives of aluminium are dangerous.

ADI   No ADI

Used in   artificial milk, table salt

556 Calcium aluminium silicate

Source   Occurs naturally as the semi-precious stone garnet. Grossular is the calcium aluminium garnet and comes from metamorphic environments as does andradite the calcium iron garnet. It is believed that these garnets form from the metamorphic form of old deposits of siliceous limestone.

Function   Used as an anti-caking agent.

Properties   No adverse effects

ADI   No ADI

Used in   artificial milk, table salt, confectionery

558 Bentonite or pascalite

Source   Occurs naturally, mainly as montmorillonite, which comes from deposits of weathered volcanic ash in Wyoming, US.

Function	Used as an anti-caking agent and as a wine stabiliser. Bentonite is negatively charged and is used as slurry in wine to remove the positively charged proteins that would otherwise form a haze in white wine. It is insoluble in wine and is readily removed by filtration. It is also used as an intestinal "cleanser" as it removes heavy metals such as lead, cadmium and mercury. There is no scientific proof that bentonite purges have any benefit.
Properties	No adverse effects
ADI	No ADI
Used in	wine, table salt

559 Aluminium silicate or andalusite or chiastolite

Source	Occurs naturally as brown clay, Andalusite in a polymorphic form together with the minerals kyanite and sillimanite.
Function	Anti-caking and carrier of aromas.
Properties	No adverse effects
ADI	No ADI
Used in	aroma essences, instant coffee, milk powders, antacid

560 Potassium silicate or potassium "water glass"

Source	Naturally occurring mineral.
Function	Used as an anti-caking agent. It is not used in foods but present in sachets inside dried food material to keep them dry and crisp.
Properties	No adverse effects
ADI	No ADI

Used in   food sachets in packages of: taco shells, potato crisps, extruded savoury biscuits and snacks

570   Stearic acid or fatty acid

Source   Occurs naturally as an ester with glycerol forming fats in vegetables and animals. Manufactured by hydrolysing animal fats and also extracted from cascarilla bark.

Function   Glazing agent, foaming agent.

Properties No adverse effects. It is absorbed very slowly from the intestines with the aid of bile salts.

ADI   No ADI

Used in   artificial butter flavouring, vanilla essence, chewing gum, apple and orange waxes, confectionery

575   Glucono-δ-lactone or Glucono delta-lactone

Source   Manufactured from glucose.

Function   Used as an acidity regulator and a raising agent in baked goods. Glucono-delta-lactone breaks down gradually in water to release gluconic acid. The gradual decrease in pH that results from this reaction is ideal for slow curing of salami and "silken" gel formation of tofu.

Properties No adverse effects

ADI   No ADI

Used in   salami, tofu, gluten-free biscuits, gluten-free bread, yoghurt (bacteria free)

577   Potassium gluconate

Source   Manufactured by adding potassium hydroxide to oxidised glucose (gluconic acid). Gluconic acid is made by aerobic bacterial fermentation. Glucose can be oxidised to gluconic acid by glucose oxidase and catalase is used to remove toxic hydrogen peroxide.

Function   Used as a sodium replacement and sequestrant agent. Used to reduce excess sweetness of lactose-hydrolysed milk products. Potassium gluconate modifies taste by overcoming the bitter taste in low-energy drinks containing saccharine.

Properties   No adverse effects

ADI   No ADI

Used in   salt replacers, body building supplements, low-energy drinks

578   Calcium gluconate

Source   Manufactured by adding calcium hydroxide to oxidised glucose (gluconic acid). Gluconic acid is made by aerobic bacterial fermentation. Glucose can be oxidised to gluconic acid by glucose oxidase and catalase is used to remove toxic hydrogen peroxide.

Function   Used as an acidity regulator, firming agent, fortification agent for calcium in bread and fruit juice, sequestrant, stabiliser or thickener and as a texturing agent.

Properties   No adverse effects

ADI   No ADI

Used in   pudding powders, custard, canned vegetables (firming agent), bakery products, infant foods, bread, fruit juices

579   Ferrous gluconate

Source   Manufactured by adding ferrous hydroxide to oxidised glucose (gluconic acid). Gluconic acid is made by aerobic bacterial fermentation. Glucose can be oxidised to gluconic acid by glucose oxidase and catalase is used to remove toxic hydrogen peroxide.

Function   Used as an iron fortification agent and as a colour retention agent.

Properties No adverse effects

ADI   0–0.8 mg/kg body weight

Used in   olives, canned beans, canned peas, fortified breakfast cereals, fortified bread and fruit juices, infant foods

580   Magnesium gluconate

Source   Manufactured by adding magnesium hydroxide to oxidised glucose (gluconic acid). Gluconic acid is made by aerobic bacterial fermentation. Glucose can be oxidised to gluconic acid by glucose oxidase and catalase is used to remove toxic hydrogen peroxide.

Function   Used as a magnesium supplement in multi-vitamin and mineral tablets as it is readily absorbed in the intestines. Also used as an acidity regulatory and firming agent.

Properties No adverse effects

ADI   No ADI

Used in   mineral supplements, yeast foods, canned beans, canned peas, tofu, cottage cheese, cheese dips, infant foods

586   4-Hexylresorcinol

Source   Manufactured from benzene and phenol.

Function   Used as an antioxidant it prevents the development of melanosis (black spot) in fresh prawns and together with calcium chloride it is used to prevent enzymic browning of cut fruit such as apples and pears. It is also used as an oral antiseptic.

Properties No adverse effects

ADI   No ADI

Used in   throat lozenges (20 mg/100 gm), prawns (1 mg/kg), frozen apples and pears

600 FLAVOUR ENHANCERS

620   L-Glutamic acid

Source   Glutamic acid is the most abundant amino acid of all. Of the 22 amino acids found in nature, glutamic acid makes up 24% of the total amino acid content of food proteins. It is found in all proteins as part of the polypeptide chain, so that all food proteins contain glutamic acid and it is released from the protein by digestion in the gastrointestinal tract and absorbed into the blood. The pure form of glutamic acid is obtained by bacterial fermentations.

Function   Used as a sodium chloride replacer and flavour enhancer.

Properties No adverse effects. See monosodium glutamate (621).

ADI   0–120 mg/kg body weight. Not permitted in infant foods.

Used in   low-sodium chloride foods, soups, canned meals

621   Monosodium glutamate, MSG or Ajino moto

Source Monosodium glutamate is the sodium salt of the amino acid glutamic acid and it is the most abundant amino acid of all. In fact, of the 22 amino acids in proteins, glutamic acid averages 24% of the total amino acid content of food proteins by weight. It is found in all proteins as part of the polypeptide chain, so that all food proteins contain glutamic acid and it is released from the protein by digestion in the gastrointestinal tract and absorbed into the blood. The pure form of monosodium glutamate is obtained by bacterial fermentations using molasses as a carbon source.

Function It is very cheap and is used in Asian foods and soup stocks. MSG acts as a flavour enhancer. It particularly increases the flavours associated with meat, poultry and seafood. It was originally found in seaweed used in Japanese cooking. The Japanese call this enhanced flavour "Umami", which means "delicious". This is a taste common to a diversity of food sources including fish, meats, mushrooms, cheese and some vegetables, including tomatoes. Within these food sources, it is the synergistic combination of glutamates and 5'-nucleotides that creates the "Umami" taste. Physiologists have recently found that taste buds on the tongue can detect MSG.

MSG is used in only a few processed foods because many consumers still perceive it to be dangerous to health and it has been replaced by nucleosides, however, as mentioned earlier MSG can be found naturally in cheese, tomatoes and fish so that these foods contain natural levels of MSG. It is also found in vegetable and meat stocks and fermented sauces such as soy and oyster sauce.

Properties There has been a great deal of publicity about the use of MSG in foods. Scientific papers suggested that MSG could cause asthma, hives, stomach aches and muscle cramps in consumers (once called "Chinese restaurant syndrome" but now "MSG syndrome"). In 2004, the NSW Government brought out legislation about the deliberate addition of MSG to restaurant meals. However, Dr Len Tarasoff of the University of Western Sydney recently published research on MSG and health and using double blind methods he showed that MSG in levels ten times of that found in foods did not affect people's health. In fact, the author has published studies where he found that parmesan cheese, tomatoes and fish contain more MSG than any Asian meal. The symptoms seem to be due to amines such as histamine present in soy and oyster sauces used in cooking.

ADI   0–120 mg/kg body weight. Not permitted in infant foods.

Used in   soups, vegemite, tomato products, parmesan cheese, stocks, soy sauce, oyster sauce, flavour pouches, instant noodles, taco mixes, curry powders and pastes

622   Monopotassium L-glutamate or MPG

Source   It is the potassium sodium salt of the amino acid glutamic acid which is the most abundant amino acid of all. In fact, of the 22 amino acids in proteins glutamic acid averages 24% of the total amino acid content by weight. It is found in all proteins as part of the polypeptide chain, so that all food proteins contain glutamic acid and it is released from the protein by digestion in the gastrointestinal tract and absorbed into the blood. The pure form of monosodium glutamate is obtained by bacterial fermentations using molasses as a carbon source.

Function   It is very cheap and is used in Asian foods and soup stocks. MPG acts as a flavour enhancer. It particularly increases the flavours associated with meat, poultry and seafood. It was originally found in seaweed used in Japanese cooking. The Japanese call this enhanced flavour "Umami" which means "delicious". Physiologists have recently found that taste buds on the tongue can detect MPG.

MPG is used in only a few processed foods because many consumers still perceive it to be dangerous to health and it has been replaced by nucleosides, however, as mentioned earlier MPG can be found naturally in cheese, tomatoes and fish so that these foods contain natural levels of MPG. It is also found in vegetable and meat stocks and fermented sauces such as soy and oyster sauce.

Properties There has been a great deal of publicity about the use of MPG in foods. Scientific papers suggested that MPG could cause asthma, hives, stomach aches and muscle cramps in consumers (once called "Chinese restaurant syndrome" but now "MPG syndrome"). The published research on MSG and health can be applied to MPG which has showed that MSG in levels ten times of that found in foods did not affect people's health. In fact, the author has published studies where he found that parmesan cheese, tomatoes and fish contain more MSG than any Asian meal. The symptoms seem to be due to amines such as histamine present in soy and oyster sauces used in cooking.

ADI 0–120 mg/kg body weight. Not permitted in infant foods.

Used in soups, vegemite, tomato products, parmesan cheese, stocks, soy sauce, oyster sauce, flavour pouches, instant noodles, taco mixes, curry powders and pastes

623 Calcium glutamate

Source It is the calcium salt of the amino acid glutamic acid which is the most abundant amino acid of all.

In fact, of the 22 amino acids in proteins glutamic acid averages 24% of the total amino acid content by weight. It is found in all proteins as part of the polypeptide chain, so that all food proteins contain glutamic acid and it is released from the protein by digestion in the gastrointestinal tract and absorbed into the blood. The pure form of calcium glutamate is obtained by adding lime to glutamic acid obtained by bacterial fermentations using molasses as a carbon source.

Function   Calcium glutamate acts as a flavour enhancer. It particularly increases the flavours associated with meat, poultry and seafood. It was originally found in seaweed used in Japanese cooking. The Japanese call this enhanced flavour "Umami" which means "delicious".

Properties   The health controversies surrounding MSG can be applied to calcium glutamate. Scientific papers suggested that MSG could cause asthma, hives, stomach aches and muscle cramps in consumers (once called "Chinese restaurant syndrome" but now "MSG syndrome"). In 2004, the NSW Government brought out legislation about the deliberate addition of MSG to restaurant meals. However, Dr Len Tarasoff of the University of Western Sydney recently published research on MSG and health and using double blind methods he showed that MSG in levels ten times of that found in foods did not affect people's health. In fact the author has published studies where he found that parmesan cheese, tomatoes and fish contain more MSG than any Asian meal. The symptoms seem to be due to amines such as histamine present in soy and oyster sauces used in cooking.

ADI   0–120 mg/kg body weight. Not permitted in infant foods.

Used in   soups, vegemite, tomato products, parmesan cheese, stocks, soy sauce, oyster sauce, flavour pouches, instant noodles, taco mixes, curry powders and pastes

624   Monoammonium L-glutamate

Source   Manufactured by injecting ammonia into glutamic acid solutions.

Function   Sodium replacer in foods and flavour enhancer.

Properties See MSG (621).

ADI   0–120 mg/kg body weight

Used in   low-sodium foods, stocks

625   Magnesium glutamate

Source   Manufactured by adding magnesium oxide to a glutamic acid solution.

Function   Sodium replacer in foods and flavour enhancer.

Properties See MSG (621).

ADI   0–120 mg/kg body weight

Used in   low-sodium foods, stocks

627   Disodium 5'-guanylate

Source   Manufactured by fermentation using bacteria and then hydrolysing the DNA of the bacteria to nucleic acids followed by fractionation.

Function   Used as a flavour enhancer. Used synergistically with other nucleotides and MSG (621) It is one hundred times more potent than MSG (621) and twice as potent as disodium 5'-inosinate. It is used synergistically with MSG to enhance meat and vegetable flavours.

Properties No adverse effects. Naturally occurring nucleotides in the diet (up to 2 g/person/day) greatly exceeds their intake resulting from use as flavour enhancers (maximum = 4 mg/person/day). Not permitted in infant foods.

ADI No ADI

Used in sauces, curries, stock cubes and powders, soups, savoury snacks, flavoured chips, gravies, soy sauce, oyster sauce

631 Disodium 5'-inosinate

Source Manufactured by fermentation using bacteria and then hydrolysing the DNA of the bacteria to nucleic acids followed by fractionation.

Function Flavour enhancer. Used synergistically with other nucleotides and MSG (621). Its flavour enhancement is fifty times more potent than MSG.

Properties No adverse effects. Naturally occurring nucleotides in the diet (up to 2 g/person/day) greatly exceeds their intake resulting from use as flavour enhancers (maximum = 4 mg/person/day). Not permitted in infant foods.

ADI No ADI

Used in sauces, curries, stock cubes and powders, soups, savoury snacks, flavoured chips, gravies, soy sauce, oyster sauce

635 Disodium 5'-ribonucleotides

Source Manufactured by fermentation using bacteria and then hydrolysing the DNA of the bacteria to nucleic acids followed by fractionation.

Function   Flavour enhancer. Used with other nucleotides and MSG (621).

Properties   No adverse effects. Naturally occurring nucleotides in the diet (up to 2 g/person/day) greatly exceeds their intake resulting from use as flavour enhancers (maximum = 4 mg/person/day). Not permitted in infant foods.

ADI   No ADI

Used in   sauces, curries, stock cubes and powders, soups, savoury snacks, flavoured chips, gravies, soy sauce, oyster sauce

636   Maltol

Source   Naturally occurring in roasted malt and the bark of fir and lark trees from which it is extracted with petroleum ether. It is also made synthetically by fusing the sugars maltose and lactose.

Function   Used as a flavour enhancer, particularly for fruit and "caramel-like" flavours. Maltol is used to enhance sweetness intensity. In soft drinks and cordials, 15 ppm of maltol allows a sugar reduction of 10% with no loss of perceived sweetness. The more expensive ethyl maltol is four times more effective in affecting sweetness in soft drinks.

Properties   No adverse effects. Maltol is a powerful bactericide and fungicide.

ADI   0–1 mg/kg body weight

Used in   chocolate, coffee, confectionery, vanilla essence, baked products, nut products, artificial maple syrup, coffee flavour

637   Ethyl maltol

Source   Manufactured by mixing ethylation maltol with ethyl alcohol in the presence of sulphuric acid.

Function   Used as a flavour enhancer in sweet foods. Ethyl maltol can be used to enhance sweetness intensity. It is four times more effective than maltol, but it is more expensive than maltol. In soft drinks and cordials, 15 ppm of maltol can allow a sugar reduction from 38% with no loss of perceived sweetness.

Properties No adverse effects

ADI   0–2 mg/kg body weight

Used in   soft drinks, chocolate, coffee, confectionery, vanilla essence, baked products, nut products, artificial maple syrup, coffee flavour

640   Glycine or amino acetic acid

Source   Manufactured by fermentation using bacteria fermentation on molasses.

Function   Used as a flavour enhancer or sweetener, in combination with alanine or citric acid, vinegar, fruit juice, salted vegetables and sweet chilli sauce to enhance flavours.

Properties No adverse effects

ADI   No ADI

Used in   soft drinks, alcoholic mixed drinks (wine coolers and cocktails), beer, margarine, instant noodles, vinegar, peanut butter, sauces

641   L-Leucine

Source   Manufactured by fermentation using bacteria fermentation on molasses.

Function   Used as a flavour enhancer in conjunction with aspartame in sugar free or reduced foods.

Properties   No adverse effects

ADI   No ADI

Used in   diet colas, artificial sweeteners

900 FOOD GLAZINGS AND COATINGS (EDIBLE FILMS)

Vegetables and fruits are usually coated with edible films (beeswax, carnauba wax, petroleum jelly and shellac) to prevent enzymic browning and dehydration, slow down ripening, prevention of brown spots on bananas and reduce bruising during transport and handling. Confectionery is also glazed with edible coatings to give a smooth and shiny, attractive appearance. These coatings are sprayed onto the food with anti-foaming agents (1505 or 1525) which allow for a more shiny appearance.

900a   Polydimethylsiloxane or Dimethylpolysiloxane or dimethicone

Source   Manufactured from silicon dioxide and dimethylsiloxane.

Function   Used as an anti-caking agent, anti-foaming agent and emulsifier.

Properties   No adverse effects

ADI   0–1.5 mg/kg body weight (only for polymers of Polydimethylsiloxane with a molecular weight between 200 and 300).

Used in   margarine (5 gm/kg), edible oils, thickened cream, dry cake and muffin mixes, gravy mixes, curry powders, milk powders, custard powders, fruit juices, fruit nectars

901   Beeswax, white and yellow

Source   Naturally occurring. It is extracted as a by-product of the honey industry (honeycomb).

Function   Used as a glazing agent on fruit and confectionery.

Properties No adverse effects. Beeswax passes unchanged through the gastrointestinal tract.

ADI   No ADI

Used in   confectionery (500 mg/kg in total with carnauba wax), waxed fruit (250 mg/kg in total with carnauba wax)

903   Carnauba wax

Source   Naturally occurring as the protective wax on leaves of the Carnauba fan palm in South East Asia. Leaves are removed individually from the tree then cut, shredded and dried so that the wax flakes off. A kilogram of wax is obtained from about 45 leaves.

Function   Used as a glazing agent.

Properties No adverse effects

ADI   No ADI

Used in   confectionery (500 mg/kg in total with carnauba wax), waxed fruit (250 mg/kg in total with carnauba wax)

904   Shellac, "confectioner's glaze"

Source   Occurs naturally as a resin which is secreted by the female, mite-sized beetle, *Laccifer lacca*, as a protection from predator birds and as a means to hold its eggs to the bark of a tree, usually a *Ficus benjamina* cultivated for this purpose in India or Thailand. The shellac resin is extracted and bleached so that it is a colourless powder soluble in organic solvents.

Function   Used as a glazing agent on fruit and confectionery.

Properties   No adverse effects. The organic solvents that shellac is dissolved in evaporate on drying and do not remain in the foods.

ADI   No ADI

Used in   confectionery (maximum allowed 1 mg/kg in total with other permitted glazes, beeswax (901) and carnauba wax (903)), fruit (maximum allowed 250 gm/kg in total with other permitted glazes, beeswax (901) and carnauba wax (903))

905b   Petrolatum or petroleum jelly

Source   Fractionated from mineral oil.

Function   Used as a glazing agent, anti-foam agent and sealant that protects flavours and vitamins from oxidation.

Properties   No adverse effects. In excess, petroleum jelly can prevent fat soluble vitamins (A,D,E and K) from being absorbed in the small intestine. It can also cause diarrhoea.

ADI   No ADI

Used in   dried fruit and vegetables (maximum permissible 3 gm/kg), confectionery (maximum permissible 2 gm/kg), packaging (grease proof paper)

914   Oxidised polyethylene

Source   Manufactured by oxidising polyethylene with singlet oxygen. Polyethylene was first made by Hans von Pechmann, a German chemist, in 1898, who synthesised it by accident while heating diazomethane. Polyethylene is commercially manufactured now by polymerisation of ethene. It can be produced through radical polymerisation or anionic polymerisation and cationic polymerisation.

Function   Used as a humectant, packaging adhesive and wax coating.

Properties   No adverse effects

ADI   No ADI

Used in   packaging adhesive, dried fruit, confectionery, apples, pears, oranges, humectant sachets in dried foods

920   L-Cysteine monohydrochloride

Source   Synthesised from cystine found in hydrolysed keratin protein found in feathers and hair (human hair in China).

Function   Used as a raising agent in bread flour. It reduces mixing time and makes the dough more extensible and easier to work with by converting the thiol groups to disulphide groups which make up the elasticity of gluten strands and increase loaf volume.

Properties   No adverse effects. L-cysteine is an essential amino acid.

ADI   No ADI

Used in   matzah (unleavened bread), bread, bread-making flour

941   Nitrogen

Source   Manufactured by removing oxygen from air at very low temperatures (-196°C).

Function   Used as a propellant and modified atmosphere gas. Nitrogen prevents fruit ripening and protects fruit, wine, beer, stout (A ping-pong ball-like "rocket widget" is added to the product during the canning phase at the brewery. The widget ball contains nitrogen (N2). When the can is opened, the valve inside the widget is broken and nitrogen gas is released into the beer, forming a finely-bubbled, beautiful head. The widget ball is found in Kilkenny and Guinness beer cans) Also nitrogen prevents vegetables from oxidation and bacterial and mould spoilage.

Properties No adverse effects

ADI No ADI

Used in beer, wine, packaged fruit, packaged vegetables

942 Nitrous oxide or "laughing gas"

Source Manufactured by the thermal decomposition of ammonium nitrate.

Function Used as a propellant.

Properties No adverse effects. It is used as an anaesthetic in medicine and dentistry.

ADI No ADI

Used in whipped cream, beer

943a Butane

Source Manufactured from petroleum.

Function Used as a propellant for cooking oil sprays and water/oil emulsion sprays used in cooking to prevent foods sticking to cookware.

Properties No adverse effects

ADI No ADI

Used in   non-stick cooking oil sprays

943b   Isobutane

Source   Manufactured from petroleum.

Function   Used as a propellant for cooking oil sprays and
               water/oil emulsion sprays used in cooking to
               prevent foods sticking to cookware.

Properties No adverse effects

ADI   No ADI

Used in   non-stick cooking oil sprays

944   Propane

Source   Manufactured from petroleum.

Function   Used as a propellant for cooking oil sprays and water/
               oil emulsion sprays used in cooking to prevent foods
               sticking to cookware.

Properties No adverse effects

ADI   No ADI

Used in   non-stick cooking oil sprays

946   Octafluorocyclobutane

Source   Manufactured from petroleum.

Function   Used as a propellant for cooking oil sprays and water/
               oil emulsion sprays used in cooking to prevent foods
               sticking to cookware.

Properties No adverse effects

ADI   No ADI

Used in   non-stick cooking oil sprays

950 Acesulphame potassium

Source Synthesised by methylation of oxathiazin dioxide and crystallisation to obtain pure acesulphame (6-methyl-1,2,3-oxathiazin-4(3H)-one-2.2-dioxide). The potassium salt is obtained by adding potassium hydroxide to this.

Function Used as an artificial sweetener. It is between 150 and 200 times sweeter than table sugar.

Properties No adverse effects. The artificial sweeteners have been under attack by Internet groups who suggest that they are all dangerous to health. However, there have been no adverse health findings and over 100 peer-reviewed scientific published studies have shown that acesulphame is perfectly safe at the concentrations used in foods, taking into account the heavy consumers such as diabetics. JECFA in 1991 concluded that acesulphame potassium does not exhibit genotoxicity or carcinogenicity. The committee also reviewed extensive toxicological studies on the breakdown products, acetoacetamide and acetoacetamide-N-sulfonic acid, which indicated that these compounds have low toxicity and are not mutagenic. Based on the reviewed data and a long-term rat study.

ADI 0–15 mg/kg body weight

Used in chewing gum, instant coffee, instant tea, puddings, ice cream, confectionery, preserved fruits and vegetables, milk products, baked goods, beverages

951 Aspartame

Source Synthesised from the amino acids phenylalanine and aspartic acid.

Function Used as an artificial sweetener. It is 200 times sweeter than table sugar but contains one-sixteenth of the energy (kilojoules) of table sugar.

Properties   No adverse effects. Despite many Internet sites suggesting that aspartame will give you everything from headaches to brain tumours, there is no scientific study in peer-reviewed journals that show health problems. Studies in animals have revealed that aspartame is rapidly digested to three parts, phenylalanine, aspartic acid, and the methyl ester, which are then absorbed, metabolised by the liver and kidneys, and excreted by normal biochemical pathways. A wide range of toxicological studies (acute, subchronic, chronic, teratology and genotoxicity) have been performed in various animal species. No significant toxicological or carcinogenic effect has been attributable to aspartame administration in doses up to 13 g/kg in subchronic studies (mice, hamsters, rats, dogs and monkeys) and up to 8 g/kg in chronic studies (mice and rats). Similar toxicological profiles have been undertaken on diketopiperazine (DKP), a major decomposition product of aspartame, that have shown no adverse effects attributable to DKP at doses up to 3 g/kg.

National Food Authority (NFA) investigated the consumption patterns in the general Australian population of eight food groups containing artificial sweeteners. "For a selected subgroup of high consumers of these products, estimated intakes of the four most commonly available intense sweeteners (aspartame, saccharin, cyclamate and acesulphame potassium) were compared with ADIs. For consumers of aspartame, intakes were low compared to the ADIs (7% ADI). At the extreme end of the range of intake (90th percentile intake for high consumer subgroup), reported aspartame intakes were less than 30% of the ADI."

ADI   0–40 mg/kg body weight

Used in   Typical usage concentrations in various products, aspartame-acesulphame concentration (concentrations for good manufacturing practices): beverages (190–260 ppm), desserts/dairy (380–400 ppm), chewing gum (2,600 ppm), hard candy (1,000 ppm), chocolate (800 ppm), tabletop sweeteners (10 mg/tablet)

952   Calcium cyclamate or sodium cyclamate or cyclamate

Source   Manufactured by adding lime or caustic soda respectively to cyclohexylsufamate (cyclamate).

Function   Used as an artificial sweetener. It is 40 times sweeter than table sugar but it has no energy content, or "bitter" taste that saccharine has. It is highly stable to heat, acid and alkaline. It is soluble in hot water.

Properties No adverse effects. It is excreted unchanged from the kidneys.

ADI   0–11 mg/kg body weight

Used in   soft drinks, diabetic foods, low-energy foods

953   Isomalt

Source   Manufactured from sugar beet. Equi-molar mixture of α-D-glucopyranosido-1, 6-sorbitol (GPS) (sometimes called α-D-glucopyranosido-1, 6-glucitol) and α-D-glucopyranosido-1,6-mannitol.

Function   Used as a humectant, sweetener, bulking agent and anti-caking agent. It has the same sweetness as sugar but only half the energy and it has a very low glycemic index which makes it highly suitable for diabetics and consumers on a low-energy diet. Isomalt also does not cause tooth decay.

Properties   No adverse effects. It is metabolised to glucose (50%), sorbitol (25%), and mannitol (25%).

ADI   0–25 mg/kg body weight

Used in   low-energy foods, confectionery, ice cream, desserts, cake fillings, chewing gum

954   Saccharin or calcium saccharin or sodium saccharine or potassium saccharine

Source   Manufactured from coal by-products.

Function   Used as an artificial sweetener, but has a "bitter" after taste. Usually used in conjunction with aspartame ("equal"). It is between 200 and 700 times sweeter than table sugar but has no energy content.

Properties   In 1977, after a study found it caused bladder cancer in rats, all products that contained saccharin were required to be labelled with the following statement: "Use of this product may be hazardous to your health. This product contains saccharin which has been determined to cause cancer in laboratory animals." Studies have followed diabetics who have used saccharin for years and have yet to show an increase in the incidence of bladder cancer. On 15 May 2000, the US government released a report on things known to cause cancer. When the list came out, it "de-listed" saccharin from the list of suspected carcinogens.

ADI   0–2.5 mg/kg body weight

Used in   soft drinks, diabetic foods, low-energy foods, chewing gum, confectionery

955   Sucralose or "Splenda"

Source   Manufactured from sucrose sugar by selectively replacing three hydroxy groups on the sugar molecule with three chlorine atoms.

Function   It has the 600 times the sweetness of sugar but only one fifth the energy and it has a very low glycemic index which makes it highly suitable for diabetics and consumers on a low-energy diet. Sucralose does not cause tooth decay and is stable to high processing temperatures and low pH of acid foods. It stimulates the growth of probiotic bacteria in the small intestine.

Properties   No adverse effects

ADI   0–15 mg/kg body weight

Used in   desserts, mixes, toppings, fillings, frozen dairy products, confectionery, baking mixes, breakfast cereals, nutritional foods (diet food, sport food, dairy etc.), ready meals and instant foods, savoury sauces and seasonings

956   Alitame

Source   Manufactured from the two amino acids L-aspartic acid and D-alanine.

Function   Alitame is 2,000 times sweeter than table sugar. It is permitted for use at a maximum level of 40–300 mg/kg in a wide range of foods and beverages, including bakery wares, water-based flavoured drinks, dairy-based drinks, dairy-based desserts, cream, edible ices, jams, confectionery and some dietetic foods. It is permitted for use within good manufacturing practice in table-top sweeteners and in some sugars (brown) and syrups (maple). The permitted uses in the Joint Food Standards Code of Australia and New Zealand, which was provided to the Committee, largely overlap with those in the Codex draft GSFA but also include use in flour products (including noodles and pasta), some processed fruit and vegetables, custard, jelly, sauces and toppings. In contrast, the Joint Food Standards Code allows its use only in specific bakery wares, not including bread (Australia New Zealand Food Authority, 2002).

Properties   No adverse effects.

ADI   0–1 mg/kg body weight

Used in   beverages, sugar substitutes, cold desserts, candy, baked goods, jams, jelly, sweet spreads and preserves, flour products (including noodles and pasta), processed fruit and vegetables, custard, sauces and toppings

957   Thaumatin

Source   Manufactured from proteins that have strong disulphide bonds by water extraction of the arils of the fruit of the West African perennial plant *Thaumatococcus daniellii*.

Function   Used as a flavour enhancer and sweetener (2,000 times sweeter than table sugar). It does not cause teeth decay and enhances many fruit flavours. It is stable to heat and pH. It works synergistically with other sweeteners. It has a delayed sweet taste and the sweetness persists for several minutes. It stimulates the growth of probiotic bacteria in the small intestine.

Properties   No adverse effects. A World Health Organisation review of the biologic, toxicologic, teratogenic, and allergenic, and some studies of this sweetener in humans suggest that thaumatin is not toxic. Consumption of large amounts may have a laxative effect.

ADI   No ADI

Used in   soft drinks, fruit juice, low-energy foods, confectionery, wine coolers, alcoholic fruit cordial mixers, nutritional foods (diet food, sport food, dairy etc.), ready meals and instant foods, savoury sauces and seasonings

961 Neotame or dimethyl aspartame

Source Manufactured by methylation of the dipeptide sweetener aspartame (aspartyl phenylalanine).

Function Used as an artificial sweetener and taste enhancer. Neotame is very stable in the dried form but in low pH foods it is stable for only two to three months, which is suitable for most products such as drinks and yoghurt. Neotame masks off flavours found in soy products. It also prolongs sweetness and flavour in chewing gum.

Properties No adverse effects

ADI No ADI

Used in dry low-energy drink mixes, yoghurt, diet soft drinks, ice cream, confectionery, soy milk, chewing gum, nutritional foods (diet food, sport food, dairy etc.), ready meals and instant foods, savoury sauces and seasonings

965 Maltitol and maltitol syrup or hydrogenated glucose syrup

Source Manufactured by hydrogenation of D-maltose, a sugar obtained from starch.

Function Used as a sweetener, stabiliser, emulsifier and humectant in food products. It is used to replace sucrose on a one-to-one basis but it is only 75% as sweet as sucrose. However, it contains half of the energy of sucrose. Other artificial sweeteners are usually added in formulating products. It stimulates the growth of probiotic bacteria in the small intestine.

Properties No adverse effects. Once maltitol is absorbed it is converted to energy by a metabolism that requires little or no insulin. Some of the sugar alcohol is not absorbed into the blood and is passed out of the small intestine and fermented by bacteria in the large intestine. Thus, over-consumption may produce abdominal gas and discomfort in some individuals. It does not cause tooth decay. Consumption of large amounts may have a laxative effect.

ADI No ADI

Used in chewing gum, baked products, chocolate, diet soft drinks, hard candy, ice cream, dusting powder for chewing gum, nutritional foods (diet food, sport food, dairy etc.), ready meals and instant foods, savoury sauces and seasonings

966 Lactitol or galacto-pyranosyl glucitol

Source Manufactured by reducing the glucose part of the disaccharide lactose with hydrogen and nickel.

Function Used as an artificial sweetener and humectant. Lactitol contains only half the energy as sucrose but it is only 40% as sweet. It is used together with other more intense artificial sweeteners. It is a bulking agent in low-energy foods. It stimulates the growth of probiotic bacteria in the small intestine. It does not cause tooth decay.

Properties No adverse effects. Once lactitol is absorbed it is converted to energy by a metabolism that requires little or no insulin. Some of the sugar alcohol is not absorbed into the blood and is passed out of the small intestine and fermented by bacteria in the large intestine. Thus, over-consumption may produce abdominal gas and discomfort in some individuals. Consumption of large amounts may have a laxative effect.

ADI   No ADI

Used in   chocolate, baked goods, hard and soft confectionery, frozen desserts, dusting powder for chewing gum, acidified food (cheese, pickles, salads and dressings), beverages (alcoholic and non-alcoholic), meat and poultry products, nutritional foods (diet food, sport food, dairy etc.), ready meals and instant foods, savoury sauces and seasonings

967   Xylitol

Source   Manufactured by reducing the glucose part of the disaccharide xylose with hydrogen and nickel.

Function   Used as an artificial sweetener, stabiliser and humectant. Xylitol contains only half the energy of sucrose and it has the same sweetness as sucrose. It is a bulking agent in low-energy foods. It stimulates the growth of probiotic bacteria in the small intestine. It does not cause tooth decay.

Properties   No adverse effects. Once xylitol is absorbed it is converted to energy by a metabolism that requires little or no insulin. Some of the sugar alcohol is not absorbed into the blood and is passed out of the small intestine and is fermented by bacteria in the large intestine. Thus, over consumption may produce abdominal gas and discomfort in some individuals. Consumption of large amounts may have a laxative effect.

ADI   No ADI

Used in   chocolate, baked goods, hard and soft confectionery, frozen desserts, dusting powder for chewing gum, acidified food (cheese, pickles, salads and dressings), beverages (alcoholic and non-alcoholic), meat and poultry products, nutritional foods (diet food, sport food, dairy etc.)

968   Erythritol

Source   Manufactured by reducing the glucose part of the
                 disaccharide erythrose with hydrogen and nickel.

Function   Used as an artificial sweetener and humectant.
                 Erythritol contains only one-sixtieth (1 kJ/gm) of
                 the energy of sucrose but it is only 80% as sweet. It
                 is used together with other more intense artificial
                 sweeteners. It is a bulking agent in low-energy
                 foods. It stimulates the growth of probiotic bacteria
                 as an humectant and is used in baked goods,
                 confectionery, low-energy foods and carbohydrate
                 modified foods, preventing the foods from taking
                 up water from the atmosphere and making them
                 "sticky".

Properties   No adverse effects. Once erythritol is absorbed it is
                 converted to energy by a metabolism that requires
                 little or no insulin. Some of the sugar alcohol is not
                 absorbed into the blood and is passed out of the
                 small intestine and is fermented by bacteria in the
                 large intestine. Thus, over consumption may produce
                 abdominal gas and discomfort in some individuals.
                 Consumption of large amounts may have a laxative
                 effect. Foods containing erythritol must have the
                 mandatory statement "EXCESS CONSUMPTION MAY
                 HAVE A LAXATIVE EFFECT" on the label.

ADI   No ADI

Used in   chocolate, baked goods, confectionery, frozen
                 desserts, dusting powder for chewing gum, acidified
                 food (cheese, pickles, salads and dressings), beverages
                 (alcoholic and non-alcoholic), meat and poultry
                 products, nutritional foods (diet food, sport food,
                 dairy etc.)

1001   Choline salts (acetate, chloride, carbonate and tartrate)

Source   Manufactured from soy beans by extraction of lecithin and then hydrolysis with acetic, carbonic, tartaric or hydrochloric acids. Choline is a natural component of plants and meat. It is necessary for cell structures, brain, heart, liver and nerve development. Choline is found in egg yolk, meat, liver, cereals. Best sources are foods with high fat and high cholesterol content.

Function   Used as an emulsifier.

Properties   No adverse effects. Choline reduces plasma cholesterol and is important in adequate growth and functioning of body organs.

ADI   No ADI

Used in   infant foods (9500 mg/kg), food supplements, health foods, margarine, mayonnaise, baked products, confectionery

1100 ENZYMES

Enzymes have many uses in food production. They can maximise juice extraction of pectin-rich fruits, clarify wine, break down barley for beer production or to extend shelf life in baked goods through slowing starch retrogradation. Indeed, there are hundreds of commercial brands and even more variations among each class of enzymes based on their side activities. In nature, there are thousands of enzymes and a few laboratory made enzymes customised through genetic engineering to suit a specific food processing requirement. It has been estimated fewer than 4% of the more than 12,000 enzymes known to scientists have been commercially adapted for food. Enzymes with proven food applications can save time and reduce costs. Enzymes catalyse chemical reactions without the use of high temperatures, physical force or chemicals that may produce unnecessary additives. Enzyme reactions occur at the cellular level; enzymes are viewed as functional aids to processing and not as ingredients. Enzyme activity can be chosen for a specific objective of the food manufacturing. Enzymes are proteins, so that some individuals may have an allergy to foods containing these additives. There is an additional environmental benefit through reducing energy consumption and waste from the food production plants.

1100   α-amylase

Source   Manufactured by fermentation of *Aspergillus flavus* fungi or the bacteria *Bacillus subtilis* and *Bacillus amyloliquefaciens* followed by salt extraction of the enzyme.

Function   Used as a bread improver and as an enzyme that converts starch to glucose. It is also used to partially digest starch to small molecular weight polysaccharides (enzyme modified starch). One interesting application is to add α-amylase to the hard starch gel centre of chocolates and hydrolysis of the starch produces a soft sweet centred chocolate.

Properties No adverse effects

ADI   No ADI

Used in   bread-making, glucose syrups, beer, apple juice, soft-centre chocolates

1101   Proteases (papain or bromelain or ficin)

Source   Manufactured by extraction from plants (paw paw, pineapples, fig tree sap), fungi and animals (rennet (mainly chymosin) is extracted from the fourth stomach (abomasum) of unweaned calves).

Function   Used as an aid in food processing. Papain is used as a meat tenderiser by hydrolysing tough fibres of meat tissue. Rennet is used to produce curds and whey in milk during cheese-making. Proteases are also used in the baking industry. Where appropriate, dough may be prepared more quickly if its gluten is partially hydrolysed. A heat-labile fungal protease is used so that it is inactivated early in the subsequent baking.

Properties No adverse effects

ADI No ADI

Used in meat products, cheese, baked goods

1102   Glucose oxidase

Source Manufactured by extracting the enzyme from fungi *Aspergillus niger* and *Penicillium* grown on molasses.

Function Used as an antioxidant. Glucose oxidase and catalase is a very powerful oxygen-scavenging system in packaged foods and beverages. Glucose oxidase catalyses the oxidation of glucose to glucono-1, 5-lactone and this immediately breaks down to gluconic acid using molecular oxygen and releasing hydrogen peroxide. It is used to remove either glucose or oxygen from foodstuffs in order to improve their storage capability. Hydrogen peroxide is an excellent antimicrobial agent. It sterilises the food and then it is removed by adding the enzyme catalase which transforms it to molecular oxygen and water. It is effective over the pH range 2 to 8 and is stable to temperatures up to 50°C.

Properties No adverse effects

ADI No ADI

Used in dry foods, peanuts, cashews, breakfast cereals, dried egg powder

1104   Lipases

Source   Manufactured by fermentation of fungi *Aspergillus niger*, *Aspergillus oryzae*, (which carries the gene coding for a lipase isolated from *Rhizomucor miehei*) or *Chaetomium erraticum*.

Function   Used as an enzyme to hydrolyse fats to glycerol and fatty acids to produce flavours in foods such as cheese. In the baking industry, lipase modifies both polar and non-polar flour lipids. The modified polar lipids increase the stability of gas cells in dough thus improving the bread volume and stability of the dough. Lipase is used in the oil industry to interesterify lipids and fatty acids to produce new fats that have desirable properties such as removal of trans-fats that cause heart disease. Lipases are also used in detergents to dissolve fats on equipment.

Properties   No adverse effects. If the lipase is derived from *Aspergillus oryzae*, which carries the gene coding for a lipase isolated from *Rhizomucor miehei*, then the food that contains this enzyme must be labelled as "Contains enzyme (1104) which is genetically modified".

ADI   No ADI

Used in   baked products, cooking oils, detergents, cheese, margarine, snack foods

1105   Lysozyme

Source   Extracted from bacteria that have been implanted with the human gene that synthesises lysozyme in the tear duct.

Function   Used as a wide spectrum anti-microbial that dissolves bacterial cell wall.

Properties   No adverse effects. Lysozyme is the natural antimicrobial enzyme that naturally occurs in human tears.

ADI No ADI

Used in wine, fruit juices

1200 Polydextrose

Source Manufactured by randomly bonding sorbitol to glucose. This is done in a double barrel extruder at 200°C and a condensation polymer of glucose, containing minor amounts of bound sorbitol is formed. Citric acid is used as a catalyst.

Function Used as a bulking agent and dietary fibre. Polydextrose contains only 4.2 kilojoules per gram compared to 16.5 kilojoules per gram for sugar. Polydextrose can only be partially digested. It is stable to heat and pH. It can be used to replace sugar, starch and fat in low-energy foods. It adds body, texture and mouth feel to foods.

Properties No adverse effects. Polydextrose is a carbohydrate that is resistant to digestion and absorption in the human small intestine and undergoes partial fermentation in the large intestine and promotes the beneficial physiological effects of laxation and modulation of blood glucose as well as other effects commonly associated with dietary fibre.

Polydextrose has no significant effect on blood biochemistry. In a recent publication, ingestion of 12 g polydextrose plus 50 g glucose resulted in a glycemic index of 89% (compared with a glycemic index of 100% after ingestion of 50 g glucose). Bowel function (frequency and ease of defecation) improved significantly and there were no reports of abdominal distension, abdominal cramps, diarrhoea or hypoglycaemia. Faecal weight (wet and dry) increased and faecal pH decreased proportionally to polydextrose intake. Short-chain fatty acid production notably that of butyrate, isobutyrate, and acetate is increased with polydextrose ingestion. There were substantial changes in faecal anaerobes after polydextrose intake. Bacteroides species (*B. fragilis*, *B. vulgatus*, and *B. intermedius*) decreased, whereas *Lactobacillus* and *Bifidobacterium* species increased. The caecal mucosa whole-crypt labelling index increased, with colonocyte proliferation mainly occurring in base compartments, which provided an indirect confirmation of butyrate production in the colon.

ADI   No ADI

Used in   low-energy foods, yoghurt, confectionery, chocolate, ice cream, bread, muesli bars

1201   Polyvinylpyrrolidone or PVP

Source   Manufactured by polymerising Pyrrolidone Carboxylic Acid with gamma rays.

Function   Used as a stabiliser and thickener. It is used as a bulking agent for artificial sweeteners and food dyes.

Properties No adverse effects

ADI   0–50 mg/kg body weight

Used in   table top sweeteners, food dyes

1202   Polyvinylpolypyrrolidone or PVPP

Source   Manufactured by polymerising Pyrrolidone Carboxylic Acid with gamma rays and repolymerising this product (PVP) with a free radical catalyst.

Function   Inert white powder that is insoluble in water and most organic solvents. It is used to remove bitter polyphenols from fruit juice and wine. It also removes flavour compounds so that trial runs must be carried out to ascertain the correct dosage of PVPP to be used.

Properties   No adverse effects

ADI   No ADI

Used in   wine, fruit juices, cider

1400 MODIFIED STARCHES

Starches have a molecular weight of one million. They are large polymers of glucose that can be modified by heat, acid, alkali or chemical addition of functional groups on the hydroxyl groups. Modified starches represent an intermediate stage in the normal enzymatic digestion of food starch in the human body. They are used as stabilisers and thickeners which improves mouth feel (body, smoothness, creaminess). They have a low temperature stability and long shelf life. They prevent syneresis ("splitting" or separation of aqueous and fat phases in food). Modified starches are stable at high temperatures, high shear forces and acid conditions. They can form clear viscous solutions that are ideal for sauces. Low temperature stability increases with the chemically modified starches. Modified starches can give a good sheen and glaze to icings on cakes and gravies and sauces. They maintain moisture retention, freeze and thaw stability, form and shape stability, they have good adhesion and improve "succulence". More information of a technical nature can be found at www.foodinnovation.com.

1400   Dextrin roasted starch

Source   Manufactured by cooking and drying a starch paste on steam-heated rolls. This pre-gelatinises the starch. A starch slurry or paste is then smeared in a layer on heated rotating rolls. The dried film is scraped off and then the product is ground in a mill to the desired particle size.

Function   Used as a stabiliser and thickener. Improves mouth feel. It has low temperature stability and long shelf life. Foods made with this starch have a comparatively short shelf life.

Properties   No adverse effects. It is completely digested to glucose, so that it contains 16.5 kJ/g.

ADI   No ADI

Used in   glazes for baked goods, batters, sauces, spreads, confectionery, mock cream, canned products, frozen foods, custard, fish products, shellfish coatings, meat products (binder in sausages), soft drinks, cereal snack foods, processed cheese

1401   Acid treated starch

Source   Manufactured by partial hydrolysis of starch with either hydrochloric or phosphoric acids and then neutralised with sodium hydroxide. The resultant sodium chloride or phosphate is removed prior to drying.

Function   Used as a stabiliser and thickener.

Properties   No adverse effects. It is completely digested to glucose, so that it contains 16.5 kJ/g.

ADI   No ADI

Used in   glazes for baked goods, batters, sauces, spreads, confectionery, mock cream, canned products, frozen foods, custard, fish products, shellfish coatings, meat products (binder in sausages), soft drinks, cereal snack foods, processed cheese

1402   Alkaline treated starch

Source   Manufactured by treating starch with dilute solutions of hot sodium hydroxide or potassium hydroxide and neutralising with hydrochloric acid. The resulting sodium or potassium chloride is removed prior to drying.

Function   Used as a stabiliser and thickener.

Properties No adverse effects. It is completely digested to glucose, so that it contains 16.5 kJ/g.

ADI   No ADI

Used in   glazes for baked goods, batters, sauces, spreads, confectionery, mock cream, canned products, frozen foods, custard, fish products, shellfish coatings, meat products (binder in sausages), soft drinks, cereal snack foods, processed cheese

1403   Bleached starch

Source   Manufactured by bleaching starch with sodium hypochlorite, sodium chlorite, hydrogen peroxide, potassium permanganate, peracetic acid, or ammonium persulfate with sulphur dioxide. Interaction with the starch molecules is mild because no change occurs in the physical properties of the starch or its solution except in its colour which is white. If permanganate is used only 50 ppm manganous sulphate can be present in the final product.

Function   Used as a stabiliser and thickener.

Properties No adverse effects. It is completely digested to glucose, so that it contains 16.5 kJ/g.

ADI   No ADI

Used in   glazes for baked goods, batters, sauces, spreads, confectionery, mock cream, canned products, frozen foods, custard, fish products, shellfish coatings, meat products (binder in sausages), soft drinks, cereal snack foods, processed cheese

1404   Oxidised starch

Source   Manufactured by oxidising and degrading starch granules with sodium hypochlorite.

Function   Used as a stabiliser and thickener. Some of the glucosidic linkages in oxidised starch are ruptured during oxidation and low levels of carboxyl and carbonyl groups are introduced. The relative level of carbonyl and carboxyl groups is dependent on reaction conditions. The carboxyl groups in particular are believed to be responsible for the observed paste viscosity stability. This starch gives very clear viscous sauces such as sweet chilli sauce.

Properties   No adverse effects. It is completely digested to glucose, so that it contains 16.5 kJ/g.

ADI   No ADI

Used in   glazes for baked goods, batters, sauces (sweet chilli), spreads, confectionery, mock cream, canned products, frozen foods, custard, fish products, shellfish coatings, meat products (binder in sausages), soft drinks, cereal snack foods, processed cheese

1405   Enzyme treated starches

Source   Manufactured by treating starch solutions with amylase enzymes derived from fungi. Enzyme modification results in the production of dextrose and glucose syrups and intermediate products such as maltodextrins and gums.

Function   Used as a stabiliser and thickener. The presence of smaller molecules such as dextrose gives food a sweet taste and some of the partially hydrolysed polymers stabilise frozen foods such as ice cream, preventing ice crystals forming during frozen storage which would give foods an unpleasant texture.

Properties No adverse effects. It is completely digested to glucose, so that it contains 16.5 kJ/g.

ADI No ADI

Used in glazes for baked goods, batters, sauces, spreads, confectionery, mock cream, canned products, frozen foods, custard, fish products, shellfish coatings, meat products (binder in sausages), soft drinks, cereal snack foods, processed cheese

1410   Monostarch phosphate

Source Manufactured by treating starch with alkali orthophosphates, phosphoric acid, or alkali tripolyphosphate.

Function Used as a stabiliser and thickener. This starch is particularly useful as a "binder" in sausages.

Properties No adverse effects. It is completely digested to glucose, so that it contains 16.5 kJ/g.

ADI No ADI

Used in glazes for baked goods, batters, sauces, spreads, confectionery, mock cream, canned products, frozen foods, custard, fish products, shellfish coatings, meat products (binder in sausages), soft drinks, cereal snack foods, processed cheese

1412   Distarch phosphate

Source Manufactured by use of sodium tripolyphosphate and sodium trimetaphosphate which results in cross-linking and esterification of starch chains. The overall extent of modification is small, the residual phosphate being of the order of 0.4% phosphorus.

Function Used as a stabiliser and thickener.

Properties   No adverse effects. It is completely digested to glucose, so that it contains 16.5 kJ/g. This starch can stimulate desirable bacteria growing in the small and large intestine, thus acting as a probiotic.

ADI   No ADI

Used in   glazes for baked goods, batters, sauces, spreads, confectionery, mock cream, canned products, frozen foods, custard, fish products, shellfish coatings, meat products (binder in sausages), soft drinks, cereal snack foods, processed cheese

1413   Phosphated distarch phosphate

Source   Manufactured by treating starch with a combination of sodium tripolyphosphate and sodium trimetaphosphate which results in cross-linking and esterification of starch chains. The overall extent of modification is small, the residual phosphate being of the order of 0.4% phosphorus.

Function   Used as a stabiliser and thickener.

Properties   No adverse effects. It is completely digested to glucose, so that it contains 16.5 kJ/g. This starch can stimulate desirable bacteria growing in the small and large intestine, thus acting as a probiotic.

ADI   No ADI

Used in   glazes for baked goods, batters, sauces, spreads, confectionery, mock cream, canned products, frozen foods, custard, fish products, shellfish coatings, meat products (binder in sausages), soft drinks, cereal snack foods, processed cheese

1414   Acetylated distarch phosphate

Source   Manufactured by treating starch with 0.1%

phosphorus oxychloride and 5% acetic anhydride. Vinyl acetate may be used as an alternative acetylating agent. Maximum acetylation of the hydroxide groups of starch amounts usually to 2.5% acetyl groups.

Function Used as a stabiliser and thickener.

Properties No adverse effects. It is completely digested to glucose, so that it contains 16.5 kJ/g. This starch can stimulate desirable bacteria growing in the small and large intestine, thus acting as a probiotic.

ADI No ADI

Used in glazes for baked goods, batters, sauces, spreads, confectionery, mock cream, canned products, frozen foods, custard, fish products, shellfish coatings, meat products (binder in sausages), soft drinks, cereal snack foods, processed cheese

1420 Starch acetate esterified with acetic anhydride

Source Manufactured by treating starch granules with 8% acetic anhydride and a maximum of 0.12% adipic acid, the latter acting as cross-linking agent. The maximum number of acetyl groups introduced is 2.5%. The number of adipic cross-links does not exceed more than 1 in about 1000 glucopyranose units, or not more than 0.09% adipyl groups introduced in the starch.

Function Used as a stabiliser and thickener.

Properties No adverse effects. It is completely digested to glucose, so that it contains 16.5 kJ/g. This starch can stimulate desirable bacteria growing in the small and large intestine, thus acting as a probiotic.

ADI No ADI

Used in glazes for baked goods, batters, sauces, spreads,

confectionery, mock cream, canned products, frozen
foods, custard, fish products, shellfish coatings, meat
products (binder in sausages), soft drinks, cereal
snack foods, processed cheese

1422 Acetylated distarch adipate

Source   Manufactured by treating starch with 8% acetic
anhydride and a maximum of 0.12% adipic acid, the
latter acting as cross-linking agent. The maximum
number of acetyl groups introduced is 2.5%. The
number of adipic cross-links does not exceed more
than 1 in about 1000 glucopyranose units, or not
more than 0.09% adipyl groups introduced in the
starch.

Function   Used as a stabiliser and thickener.

Properties No adverse effects. It is completely digested to
glucose, so that it contains 16.5 kJ/g. This starch can
stimulate desirable bacteria growing in the small and
large intestine, thus acting as a probiotic.

ADI   No ADI

Used in   glazes for baked goods, batters, sauces, spreads,
confectionery, mock cream, canned products, frozen
foods, custard, fish products, shellfish coatings, meat
products (binder in sausages), soft drinks, cereal
snack foods, processed cheese

1440 Hydroxypropyl starch

Source   Manufactured by treating starch granules with
propylene oxide at levels up to 25%. The resultant
starch is usually lightly oxidized, bleached or acid
modified after etherification. Substitution may
amount to a maximum of 40 ether linkages per
100 glucopyranose units if 25%. Otherwise, four to

six ether linkages per 100 glucopyranose units if 5% propylene oxide is used.

Function Used as a stabiliser and thickener.

Properties No adverse effects. It is completely digested to glucose, so that it contains 16.5 kJ/g.

ADI No ADI

Used in glazes for baked goods, batters, sauces, spreads, confectionery, mock cream, canned products, frozen foods, custard, fish products, shellfish coatings, meat products (binder in sausage), soft drinks, cereal snack foods, processed cheese

1442 Hydroxypropyl distarch phosphate

Source Manufactured by treating tapioca starch granules with 0.1% phosphorus oxychloride and eight to 10% of propylene oxide. Cross-linkage would be no greater than is experienced on modification with phosphorus oxychloride alone and ether linkages would probably not exceed 20% 100 anhydroglucose units.

Function Used as a stabiliser and thickener.

Properties No adverse effects. It is completely digested to glucose, so that it contains 16.5 kJ/g.

ADI No ADI

Used in glazes for baked goods, batters, sauces, spreads, confectionery, mock cream, canned products, frozen foods, custard, fish products, shellfish coatings, meat products (binder in sausages), soft drinks, cereal snack foods, processed cheese

1450 Starch sodium octenylsuccinate

Source Manufactured by treating starch granules with

octenylsuccinic anhydride. The finished product has a degree of substitution of 0.02% octenyl succinic groups on the hydroxyl groups of starch.

Function   Used as a stabiliser and thickener. This starch is anionic and the negative charge it carries makes it a very good emulsifier that can be stable at low pH and high and low storage temperatures.

Properties   No adverse effects

ADI   No ADI

Used in   butter, infant foods (50 mg/kg allowed), glazes for baked goods, batters, encapsulation of flavours, sauces, spreads, confectionery, mock cream, canned products, frozen foods, custard, fish products, shellfish coatings, meat products (binder in sausages), soft drinks, cereal snack foods, processed cheese

1505   Triethyl citrate or Citrofol®

Source   Manufactured by esterifying the carboxylic groups of citric acid with ethanol. Citric acid is made by fermentation of molasses by fungi.

Function   Used as an anti-foaming agent, a carrier of flavours and as a whipping aid to egg whites (pavlova). It is also used as a sour taste enhancer in lemon squash.

Properties   No adverse effects

ADI   0–20 mg/kg body weight

Used in   soft drinks, flavours, meringues

1518   Triacetin or Glyceryl triacetate or Enzactin

Source   Manufactured by esterifying glycerol hydroxide groups with acetic acid.

Function   Used as an humectant and because it has a high solvency power and low volatility it is a good solvent and fixative for many flavours and fragrances. One of its main uses is as a plasticiser in chewing gum.

Properties   No adverse effects

ADI   No ADI

Used in   flavours, fragrances, chewing gum, pet foods

1520   Propylene glycol

Source   Manufactured from the petroleum fraction propylene. Propylene is converted into propylene oxide, either by a reaction with hypochlorous acid and neutralised with calcium hydroxide, or in a one-step reaction with hydroperoxide, ROOH, in the presence of a molybdenum or vanadium catalyst. Propylene oxide is then hydrolysed to propylene glycol.

Function   Used as a stabiliser and thickener. It is an odourless and tasteless liquid. It also protects food from freezing and helps as a preservative.

Properties   No adverse effects. The Department of Health and Human Services (DHHS), the International Agency for Research on Cancer (IARC) in the US have not classified ethylene glycol and propylene glycol for carcinogenicity. Studies with people who used ethylene glycol did not show carcinogenic effects. Animal studies also have not shown these chemicals to be carcinogens.

ADI   0–25 mg/kg body weight

Used in   pet foods (not cat food), cake mixes, salad dressings, soft drinks, popcorn, food colourings, fat-free ice cream, sour cream

1521   Polyethylene glycol 8000

Source   Manufactured by polymerisation of ethylene oxide with either water, mono ethylene glycol or diethylene glycol as starting material, under alkaline catalysis.

Function   Used as an anti-foaming agent.

Properties No adverse effects. Polyethylene glycol has been shown to suppress colon cancer.

ADI   0–10 mg/kg body weight

Used in   food lubricants, pet foods, food flavours, multi-vitamin capsules

Appendices

Additives, their functions and code numbers, in alphabetical order

Symbols used in this list:
α = alpha; β = beta; δ = delta; γ = gamma.

Acacia (thickener, stabiliser) 414

Acesulphame potassium (sweetener) 950

Acetate, *see* Choline salts (emulsifier) 1001

Acetic acid, glacial (acidity regulator) 260

Acetic and fatty acid esters of glycerol (emulsifier, stabiliser) 472a

Acetylated distarch adipate (thickener, stabiliser) 1422

Acetylated distarch phosphate (thickener, stabiliser) 1414

Acid brilliant green BS, *see* Green S (colour) 142

Acid treated starch (thickener, stabiliser) 1401

Adipic acid (acidity regulator) 355

Agar (thickener, gelling agent, stabiliser) 406

Ajino moto, *see* Monosodium glutamate (flavour enhancer) 621

Alginic acid (thickener, stabiliser) 400

Alitame (sweetener) 956

Alkaline treated starch (thickener, stabiliser) 1402

Alkanet (colour) 103

Alkannin, *see* Alkanet (colour) 103

Allo-maleic acid, *see* Fumaric

Bone phosphate
(anti-caking agent,
emulsifier) 542

Brilliant black BN
(colour) 151

Brilliant blue FCF (colour) 133

Brilliant black PN, *see*
Brilliant black BN (colour) 151

Brilliant scarlet, *see*
Ponceau 4R (colour) 124

Bromelain, *see* Proteases
(stabiliser, enzyme) 1101

Brown HT (colour) 155

Butane (propellant) 943a

Butylated hydroxyanisole
(antioxidant) 320

Butylated hydroxytoluene
(antioxidant) 321

Calcium acetate
(acidity regulator) 263

Calcium alginate
(thickener, stabiliser,
gelling agent) 404

**Calcium aluminium
silicate** (anti-caking
agent) 556

Calcium ascorbate
(antioxidant) 302

Calcium benzoate
(preservative) 213

Calcium carbonate
(colour, anti-caking agent) 170

Calcium chloride
(firming agent) 509

Calcium citrate (acidity
regulator, stabiliser) 333

Calcium cyclamate
(sweetener) 952

**Calcium disodium
EDTA,** *see* Calcium
disodium ethylene-
diaminetetraacetate
(preservative, antioxidant) 385

**Calcium disodium
ethylenediaminetetra-
acetate** (preservative,
antioxidant) 385

Calcium fumarate
(acidity regulator) 367

Calcium gluconate
(acidity regulator,
firming agent) 578

Calcium glutamate
(flavour enhancer) 623

Calcium hydroxide
(acidity regulator,
firming agent) 526

Calcium lactate
(acidity regulator) 327

Calcium lactylate
(emulsifier, stabiliser) 482

Calcium malate
(acidity regulator) 352

Calcium oleyl lactylate,
see Calcium lactylate
(emulsifier, stabiliser) 482

Calcium oxide
(acidity regulator) 529

Calcium phosphates
(acidity regulator,
emulsifier, stabiliser,
anti-caking agent) 341

Calcium propionate
(preservative) 282

Calcium saccharin, *see*
Saccharin (sweetener) 954

Calcium salts of fatty acids,
see Aluminium salts of fatty

acids (emulsifier, stabiliser,
anti-caking agent) 470

Calcium silicate
(anti-caking agent) 552

Calcium sorbate
(preservative) 203

Calcium stearoyl lactylate,
see Calcium lactylate
(emulsifier, stabiliser) 482

Calcium sulphate
(firming agent) 516

Calcium tartrate
(acidity regulator) 354

Caramel I (colour) 150a

Caramel II (colour) 150b

Caramel III (colour) 150c

Caramel IV (colour) 150d

Carbon black (colour) 153

Carbon dioxide
(propellant) 290

Carbonate, see
Choline salts (emulsifier) 1001

Carboxy benzene, see
Benzoic acid (preservative) 210

Carmine (colour) 120

Carminic acid, see
Carmines (colour) 120

Carmoisine, see
Azorubine (colour) 122

Carnauba wax
(glazing agent) 903

Carob bean gum,
see Locust bean gum
(thickener, stabiliser) 410

β-apo-8' Carotenal
(colour) 160e

β-Carotene (colour) 160a

β-apo-8' Carotenoic

acid (colour) 160f

Carrageenan
(thickener, gelling
agent, stabiliser) 407

**Cellulose microcrystalline
and powdered** (anti-
caking agent) 460

Chiastolite, see
Aluminium silicate
(anti-caking) 559

Chloride, see Choline
salts (emulsifier) 1001

Chlorophyll (colour) 140

**Chlorophyll-copper
complex** (colour) 141

Choline salts
(emulsifier) 1001

Citric acid (acidity
regulator, antioxidant) 330

**Citric and fatty acid
esters of glycerol**
(emulsifier, stabiliser) 472c

Citrofol®, see Triethyl
citrate (anti-foaming
agent) 1505

Cochineal, see Carmine
(colour) 120

Confectioner's glaze, see
Shellac (glazing agent) 904

Crocetin, see Saffron
(colour) 164

Crocin, see Saffron
(colour) 164

Cryptoxanthin, see
Kryptoxanthin (colour) 161c

Cupric sulphate
(mineral salt) 519

Curcumin (colour) 100

Cyclamate, see Calcium

cyclamate (sweetener)   952

Dextrin roasted starch
(thickener, stabiliser)   1400

Di-glycerides of fatty acids
(emulsifier, stabiliser)   471

Diacetyltartaric and fatty acid esters of glycerol
(emulsifier)   472e

Digallic Acid, *see* Tannic acid (colour, emulsifier, stabiliser, thickener)   181

Dimethicone, *see* Polydimethylsiloxane, (anti-caking agent, emulsifier)   900a

Dimethyl aspartame, *see* Neotame (sweetener, flavour enhancer)   961

Dimethyl dicarbonate
(preservative)   242

Dimethylpolysiloxane, *see* Polydimethylsiloxane (anti-caking agent, emulsifier)   900a

Dioctyl sodium sulphosuccinate
(emulsifier)   480

Disodium 5'-guanylate
(flavour enhancer)   627

Disodium 5'-inosinate
(flavour enhancer)   631

Disodium 5'-ribonucleotide
(flavour enhancer)   635

DL-Malic acid
(acidity regulator)   296

Distarch phosphate
(thickener, stabiliser)   1412

Dodecyl gallate
(antioxidant)   312

Edible calcium phosphate of bone, *see* Bone phosphate (anti-caking agent, emulsifier)   542

EDTA, *see* Calcium disodium ethylenediamine tetraacetate (preservative, antioxidant)   385

Enzactin, *see* Triacetin (humectant)   1518

Enzyme treated starches
(thickener, stabiliser)   1405

Epsom salts, *see* Magnesium sulphate (firming agent)   518

Epsomite, *see* Magnesium sulphate (firming agent)   518

Erythorbic acid
(antioxidant)   315

Erythritol (humectant, sweetener)   968

Erythrosine (colour)   127

Ethyl maltol
(flavour enhancer)   637

Fast green FCF (colour)   143

Fatty acid, *see* stearic acid (glazing agent, foaming agent)   570

Ferric ammonium citrate (acidity regulator, anti-caking agent)   381

Ferrous gluconate
(colour retention agent)   579

Ficin, *see* Proteases (stabiliser, enzyme)   1101

Flavoxanthin (one of the Xanthophylls) (colour)   161a

Food green S, *see* Green S

(colour) 142

French chalk, *see*
Magnesium silicate
(anti-caking agent) 553

Fumaric acid
(acidity regulator) 297

Galacto-pyranosyl glucitol,
see Lactitol (sweetener,
humectant) 966

Gallotannic acid, *see* Tannic
acid (colour, emulsifier,
stabiliser, thickener) 181

Gallotannin, *see* Tannic
acid (colour, emulsifier,
stabiliser, thickener) 181

Glycerite, *see* Tannic
acid (colour, emulsifier,
stabiliser, thickener) 181

Gellan gum (thickener,
stabiliser, gelling agent) 418

Glucono δ-lactone
(acidity regulator, raising
agent) 575

Glucono δ-lactone, *see*
Glucono δ-lactone (acidity
regulator, raising agent) 575

Glucose oxidase
(antioxidant) 1102

Glycerin (humectant) 422

Glycerite, *see* Tannic acid 181

Glycerol, *see* Glycerin
(humectant) 422

**Glycerol esters of wood
rosins** (emulsifier,
stabiliser) 445

Glyceryl triacetate, *see*
Triacetin (humectant) 1518

Glycine (flavour enhancer) 640

Gold (colour) 175

Grape skin, *see*
Anthocyanins (colour) 163

Green S (colour) 142

Guar gum (thickener,
stabiliser) 412

Gum Arabic, *see* Acacia
(thickener, stabiliser) 414

4-Hexylresorcinol
(antioxidant) 586

Hydrochloric acid
(acidity regulator) 507

**Hydrogenated glucose
syrup,** *see* Maltitol and
maltitol syrup (sweetener,
stabiliser, emulsifier,
humectant) 965

Hydroxypropyl cellulose
(thickener, stabiliser,
emulsifier) 463

**Hydroxypropyl distarch
phosphate** (thickener,
stabiliser) 1442

**Hydroxypropyl
methylcellulose**
(thickener, stabiliser,
emulsifier) 464

Hydroxypropyl starch
(thickener, stabiliser) 1440

Indigo carmine, *see*
Indigotine (colour) 132

Indigotine (colour) 132

Iota carageenan, *see*
Processed eucheuma
seaweed (thickener,
gelling agent, stabiliser) 407a

Irish moss, *see*
Carrageenan, (thickener,
gelling agent, stabiliser) 407

Iron oxide (colour) 172

Isobutane (propellant)　943b

Isomalt (humectant, sweetener, bulking agent, anti-caking agent)　953

Karaya gum (thickener, stabiliser)　416

Kryptoxanthin (colour)　161c

Kurkum, see Curcumin (colour)　100

Lactic acid (acidity regulator)　270

Lactic and fatty acid esters of glycerol (emulsifier, stabiliser)　472b

Lactitol (sweetener, humectant)　966

Lactoflavin, see Riboflavin (colour)　101

Larch gum, see Arabinogalactan (thickener, gelling gent, stabiliser)　409

Laughing gas, see Nitrous oxide (propellant)　942

L-Cysteine monohydrochloride (raising agent)　920

Lecithin (antioxidant, emulsifier)　322

L-Glutamic acid (flavour enhancer)　620

Lipases (enzyme)　1104

Lissamine green, see Green S (colour)　142

L-Leucine (flavour enhancer)　641

L+Sodium tartrate (acidity regulator)　335

L+Tartaric acid (acidity regulator, antioxidant)　334

Locust bean gum (thickener, stabiliser)　410

Lutein (colour)　161b

Lycopene (colour)　160d

Lysozyme (enzyme, preservative)　1105

Magnesite, see Magnesium carbonate (acidity regulator, anti-caking agent)　504

Magnesium carbonate (acidity regulator, anti-caking agent)　504

Magnesium chloride (firming agent)　511

Magnesium gluconate (acidity regulator, firming agent)　580

Magnesium glutamate (flavour enhancer)　625

Magnesium lactate (acidity regulator)　329

Magnesium oxide (anti-caking agent)　530

Magnesium phosphates (acidity regulator, anti-caking agent)　343

Magnesium salts of fatty acids, see Aluminium salts of fatty acids (emulsifier, stabiliser, anti-caking agent)　470

Magnesium silicate (anti-caking agent)　553

Magnesium sulphate (firming agent)　518

Malic acid, see DL Malic

acid (acidity regulator) 296

Maltitol and maltitol syrup (sweetener, stabiliser, emulsifier, humectant) 965

Maltol (flavour enhancer) 636

Manna sugar, *see* Mannitol,(sweetener, humectant) 421

Mannitol, (sweetener, humectant) 421

Metatartaric acid (acidity regulator) 353

Methyl cellulose (thickener, stabiliser, emulsifier) 461

Methyl ethyl ester, *see* β-apo-8' Carotenoic acid (colour) 160f

Methyl ethyl cellulose (thickener, stabiliser, emulsifier, foaming agent) 465

Methylparaben (preservative) 218

Methyl-p-hydroxy-benzoate, *see* Methylparaben (preservative) 218

Mixed tartaric, acetic and fatty acid esters of glycerol (emulsifier, stabiliser) 472f

Mono-glycerides of fatty acids (emulsifier, stabiliser) 471

Monoammonium L-glutamate (flavour enhancer) 624

Monopotassium L-glutamate (flavour enhancer) 622

Monosodium glutamate

(flavour enhancer) 621

Monostarch phosphate (thickener, stabiliser) 1410

MPG, *see* Monopotassium L-glutamate (flavour enhancer) 622

MSG, *see* Monosodium glutamate (flavour enhancer) 621

Natamycin (preservative) 235

Natrolite, *see* Sodium aluminosilicate (anti-caking agent) 554

Natural red, *see* Carmine (colour) 120

Neotame (sweetener) 961

Nisin (preservative) 234

Nitrogen (propellant) 941

Nitrous oxide (propellant) 942

Octafluorocyclobutane (propellant) 946

Octyl gallate (antioxidant) 311

Oxidised polyethylene (humectant) 914

Oxidised starch (thickener, stabiliser) 1404

Papain, *see* Proteases (stabiliser, enzyme) 1101

Paprika oleoresins (colour) 160c

Pectins (thickener, stabiliser, gelling agent) 440

Petrolatum (glazing agent) 905b

Petroleum jelly, *see* Petrolatum (glazing agent) 905b

Phosphated distarch

phosphate (thickener, stabiliser)   1413

Phosphoric acid (acidity regulator)   338

Pimaricin, *see* Natamycin (preservative)   235

Polydextrose (humectant, bulking agent, stabiliser, thickener)   1200

Polydimethylsiloxane (anti-caking agent, emulsifier)   900a

Polyethylene (40) stearate (emulsifier)   431

Polyethylene glycol 8000 (anti-foaming agent)   1521

Polyglycerol esters of fatty acids (emulsifier)   475

Polyglycerol esters of interesterified ricinoleic acid (emulsifier)   476

Polyoxyethylene (20) sorbitan monostearate, *see* Polysorbate 60 (emulsifier)   435

Polyoxyethylene (20) sorbitan tristearate, *see* Polysorbate 65 (emulsifier)   436

Polyoxyethylene (20) sorbitan mono-oleate, *see* Polysorbate 80 (emulsifier)   433

Polysorbate 60 (emulsifier)   435

Polysorbate 65 (emulsifier)   436

Polysorbate 80 (emulsifier)   433

Polyvinylpyrrolidone (stabiliser)   1202

Polyvinylpolypyrrolidone (stabiliser)   1202

Ponceau 4R (colour)   124

Potassium acetate (acidity regulator)   261

Potassium acid tartrate, *see* Potassium tartrate (acidity regulator, stabiliser)   336

Potassium adipate (acidity regulator)   357

Potassium alginate (thickener, stabiliser)   402

Potassium aluminium silicate (anti-caking)   555

Potassium ascorbate (antioxidant)   303

Potassium benzoate (preservative)   212

Potassium bisulphite (preservative)   228

Potassium carbonates (acidity regulator, stabiliser)   501

Potassium chloride (gelling agent)   508

Potassium citrate (acidity regulator, stabiliser)   332

Potassium diacetate, *see* Potassium acetate (acidity regulator)   261

Potassium ferrocyanide (anti-caking agent)   536

Potassium fumarate (acidity regulator)   366

Potassium gluconate (sequestrant)   577

Potassium hexacyano-

Sodium lactylate
(emulsifier, stabiliser)   481

Sodium malates (acidity
regulator, humectant)   350

Sodium metabisulphite
(preservative)   223

Sodium metaphosphate,
insoluble, *see* Potassium
polymetaphosphate
(emulsifier, stabiliser)   452

Sodium nitrate
(preservative, colour
fixative)   251

Sodium nitrite
(preservative, colour
fixative)   250

Sodium oleyl lactylate,
see Sodium lactylate
(emulsifier, stabiliser)   481

Sodium phosphates
(acidity regulator,
emulsifier, stabiliser)   339

Sodium polyphosphates,
glassy, *see* Potassium
polymetaphosphate
(emulsifier, stabiliser)   452

Sodium propionate
(preservative)   281

Sodium pyrophosphate,
see Potassium pyrophosphate
(emulsifiers, acidity
regulators, stabilisers)   450

Sodium saccharine, *see*
Saccharin (sweetener)   954

Sodium salts of fatty acids,
see Aluminium salts of fatty
acids (emulsifier, stabiliser,
anti-caking agent)   470

Sodium sorbate
(preservative)   201

Sodium stearoyl lactylate,
see Sodium lactylate
(emulsifier, stabiliser)   481

Sodium sulphate
(acidity regulator)   514

Sodium sulphite
(preservative)   221

Sodium tartrate (L+)
(acidity regulator)   335

Sodium tripolyphosphate,
see Potassium
tripolyphosphate
(acidity regulator)   451

Sorbic acid (preservative)   200

Sorbitan monostearate
(emulsifier)   491

Sorbitan tristearate
(emulsifier)   492

Sorbitol (sweetener,
humectant, emulsifier)   420

Sorbitol syrup, *see* Sorbitol
(sweetener, humectant,
emulsifier)   420

Splenda, *see* Sucralose
(sweetener)   955

Stannous chloride
(antioxidant)   512

**Starch acetate esterified
with acetic anhydride**
(thickener, stabiliser)   1420

**Starch sodium
octenylsuccinate**
(thickener, stabiliser)   1450

Stearic acid (glazing agent,
foaming agent)   570

Stearic fatty acid (glazing
agent, foaming agent)   570

Succinic acid
(acidity regulator)   363

Sucralose (sweetener) 955

Sucrose acetate isobutyrate
(emulsifier, stabiliser) 444

**Sucrose esters of fatty
acids** (emulsifier) 473

Sulphur dioxide
(preservative) 220

Sunset yellow 3FCF
(colour) 110

Talc, *see* Magnesium silicate
(anti-caking agent) 553

Tannic acid (colour,
emulsifier, stabiliser,
thickener) 181

Tannins, *see* Tannic acid
(colour, emulsifier,
stabiliser, thickener) 181

Tartaric acid (L+) (acidity
regulator, antioxidant) 334

Tartrate, *see* Choline
salts (emulsifier) 1001

Tartrazine (colour) 102

tert-Butylhydroquinone
(antioxidant) 319

Thaumatin (flavour
enhancer, sweetener) 957

Titanium dioxide (colour) 171

α-**Tocopherol** (antioxidant) 307

δ-**Tocopherol** (antioxidant) 309

γ-**Tocopherol** (antioxidant) 308

Tocopherols concentrate,
mixed (antioxidant) 306

Tragacanth gum
(thickener, stabiliser) 413

Triacetin (humectant) 1518

Triammonium citrate,
see Ammonium citrate
(acidity regulator) 380

Triethyl citrate
(antifoaming agent) 1505

Turmeric, *see*
Curcumin (colour) 100

Tween 60, *see*
Polysorbate 60 (emulsifier) 435

Tween 65, *see*
Polysorbate 65 (emulsifier) 436

Tween 80, *see*
Polysorbate 80 (emulsifier) 433

Vegetable carbon, *see*
Carbon black (colour) 153

Violoxanthin (colour) 161e

Vitamin B2, *see* Riboflavin
(colour) 101

Vitamin C, *see* Ascorbic
acid (antioxidant) 300

Xanthan gum (thickener,
stabiliser) 415

Xanthophylls (colour),
see Flavoxanthin 161a,
Kryptoxanthin 161c, Lutein
161b, Rhodoxanthin 161f,
Rubixanthin 161d, and
Violoxanthin 161e

Xylitol (sweetener,
humectant, stabiliser) 967

Yellow 5, *see* Tartrazine
(colour) 102

Bibliography

Abd Elmoneim, O., Elkhalifa & Abdullahi H., El-Tinay Grotz, V.L., Henry, R.R., McGill, J.B., et al. (2003). *Lack of effect of sucralose on glucose homeostasis in subjects with type 2 diabetes. Journal of the American Dietetics Association.* 103 (12), 1607–1612.

American Diabetes Association. (2004). Nutrition principles and recommendations in diabetes – Position statement. *Diabetes Care,* January.

Anderson, H.H., David, N.A. & Leake, C.D. (1931). Oral toxicity of certain alkyl resorcinols in guinea-pigs and rabbits. *Proceedings of the Society of Biological Medicine,* 28, 609–612.

Ashby, J., Tennant, R.W., Zeiger, E. & Stasiewicz, S. (1989). Classification according to chemical structure, mutagenicity to Salmonella and level of carcinogenicity of a further 42 chemicals tested for carcinogenicity by the US National Toxicology Program. *Mutation Research,* 223, 73–103.

Australia New Zealand Food Authority (2006). *Australia New Zealand Food Standards Code, Standard 1.3.1 Food Additives,* Canberra (available at www.anzfa.gov.au).

Food Standards Australia New Zealand, (2006). *Food Standards Australia New Zealand ensures safe food by developing effective food standards for Australia and New Zealand.* www.foodstandards.gov.au.

Hambridge, T. (2002a) *Information sheet for Australia on alitame.* Canberra, Australia New Zealand Food Authority. Submitted to WHO by the Australia New Zealand Food Authority.

Mezitis, N.H., Maggio, C.A., Koch, P, et al.(1996). Glycemic effect of a single high oral dose of the novel sweetener sucralose in patients with diabetes. *Diabetes Care.* 19, 1004–1005.

National Food Authority (1995). *Survey of intense sweetener consumption in Australia, Final report.* ISBN 0 642 22736 5.

Neiser, S., Draget, K. I. & Smidsrod, O. (2000). Gel formation in heat-treated bovine serum albumin-k-carrageenan systems. *Food Hydrocolloids,* 14, 95–110.

O'Brien, Nabors, Lyn (Ed) (2001). *Alternative sweeteners.* (3rd edn) Marcel Dekker, Inc. New York.

www.fda.gov. Food and Drug agency of the US (2006).

www.herbstreith-fox.de/eindex.htm. Pectin specialists, includes information and news regarding this area.

www.thegacgroup.com/. Links, images, and Ghatti gums.

Notes

Notes